DENTAL MATERIALS GUIDE

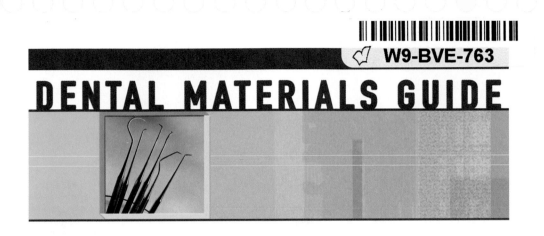

DENTAL MATERIALS GUIDE

DONNA PHINNEY

CDA, FADAA, M.Ed.
Spokane Community College

JUDY HALSTEAD

CDA, BA
Spokane Community College

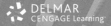

Australia   Canada   Mexico   Singapore   Spain   United Kingdom   United States

DELMAR
CENGAGE Learning·

Dental Materials Guide
by Donna Phinney and Judy Halstead

**Vice President, Career and
Professional Editorial**
Dave Garza

Director of Learning Solutions
Matthew Kane

Senior Product Manager
Darcy M. Scelsi

**Vice President, Career
and Professional Marketing**
Jennifer McAvey

Marketing Manager
Lynn Henn

Production Director
Carolyn Miller

Content Project Manager
Kenneth McGrath

Senior Art Director
Jack Pendleton

Printed in China
1 2 3 4 5 6 7 12 11 10 09 08

For product information and technology assistance, contact us at
Professional & Career Group Customer Support, 1-800-648-7450
For permission to use material from this text or product,
submit all requests online at www.cengage.com/permissions.
Further permissions questions can be e-mailed to
permissionrequest@cengage.com.

Library of Congress Control Number: 2007943969

ISBN-13: 978-1-418-05199-0
ISBN-10: 1-4180-5199-3

Delmar Cengage Learning
5 Maxwell Drive
Clifton Park, NY 12065-2919
USA

Cengage Learning products are represented in Canada by Nelson Education, Ltd.

For your lifelong learning solutions, visit delmar.cengage.com.

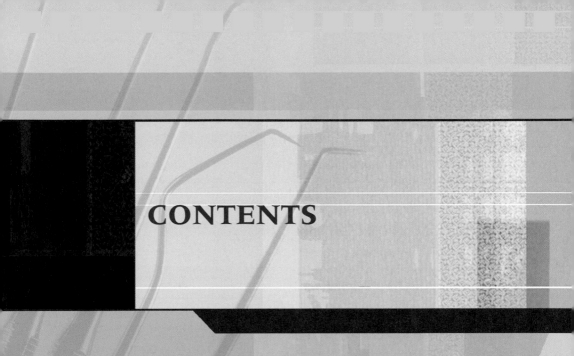

CONTENTS

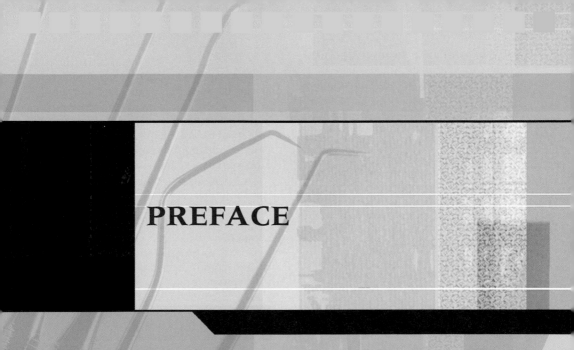

PREFACE

PREFACE FOR DENTAL MATERIALS GUIDE

There are so many different materials used in dentistry that the sheer number can be overwhelming when trying to learn the types of materials and where and when they are used.

Dental materials are continually developing and changing as technology advances and different clinical needs arise. For example many dental materials now have fluoride added to their composition for fluoride strengthens the enamel. Another change has been occurring as more and more people want the "natural" look and from this trend a number of materials are being developed for esthetic/cosmetic dentistry.

The delivery methods of many materials are also advancing. They are being made easier to prepare, mix, and place for the dentist and the dental assistant. Instead of the materials coming in a powder/liquid composition form, many materials now come in cartridges or canules for easy dispensing with a dispensing gun. Some come in automix forms with disposable mixing tips that mix the materials as they are being dispensed. There are also single dose packets available and capsules for quick mixing with little need for clean up.

The dental assistant is responsible for knowing all of the materials used in a dental office. They order, stock, prepare and mix a large variety of materials. Some states also allow the assistant to place some of the materials in the oral cavity. There are many types of materials used in the dental office; examples include materials used in dental hygiene, restorative materials or materials only used in the laboratory. Having a comprehensive grasp of the materials used is also beneficial for patient education and protection.

The *Dental Materials Pocket Guide* is designed to give the dental assistant student the basic knowledge of a variety of dental materials in each category of materials used in a dental office. This pocket guide includes materials used in specialty offices, dental hygiene, and a few materials the patient uses at home. It allows the student to see how the materials are divided into uses and then gives examples of each type. There are too many different brands of each material to include in one text but we tried to include a variety of materials for the dental assistant to gain an understanding of the basics so they can use this information and apply it to any brand name. The materials are categorized in groupings that follow basic dental procedures in general and specialty dentistry. For example, one section covers the impression materials; another section covers all the dental cements. This allows students to easily study similar information. The pocket guide covers the use, composition, properties, OSHA properties, mixing and setting times, and directions for each material.

We feel students will find this guide to be a very helpful tool in their learning process as an adjunct to their main textbook and clinic/laboratory experience.

ACKNOWLEDGEMENTS

We want to thank those who have encouraged and motivated us to develop this dental materials guide. Thanks to our students for asking us to develop a guide similar to the instrument guide for dental materials. They want better ways to learn and remember all the materials used in dentistry. Each year, student quest for knowledge becomes more creative and inventive. The need for a quick reference is necessary in the busy lives of students. Our goal was a quick reference to meet their needs.

We would like to thank Thomson Delmar Learning which is now Cengage Learning and its staff whose assistance and encouragement are greatly appreciated. We would like especially to acknowledge Kalen Conerly and Maureen Rosener, Acquisitions Editors and Darcy Scelsi, Senior Product Manager, for her dedication and guidance with this project.

As with our other projects we greatly would like to thank our husbands, Dwayne and Chuck, and our families, for their continued support through all of our endeavors.

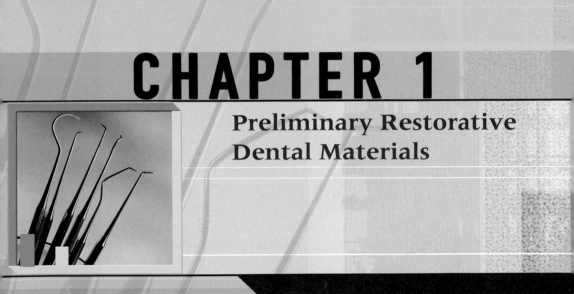

CHAPTER 1

Preliminary Restorative Dental Materials

CARIES DETECTORS/INDICATORS

Caries detectors or caries indicators are special dyes used to detect caries by distinguishing between good, sound, hard dentin, and dentin that is infected with bacteria and is softened.

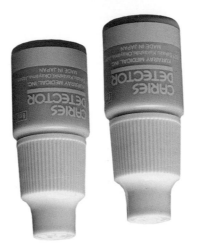

CARIES DETECTOR

MANUFACTURER:
Kuraray America, Inc.

USE:
- Identification of carious dentin
- Aids in the removal of the carious dentin layer for a conservative preparation
- Minimizes removal of remineralizable, healthy dentin, thus protecting the pulp

COMPOSITION:
- Propane-1, 2-diol with D & C Red #30 dye

PROPERTIES:
- Supplied in small bottles
- Comes in red dyes
- Must be rinsed off after a reaction time of 10 seconds
- Do not use after expiration date
- Do not store at temperature above 77 degrees F (25 degrees C)
- Avoid exposure to sunlight

OSHA PRECAUTIONS:

- Eye and skin irritation possible
- Should not be ingested
- Product is flammable. Keep away from open flame.
- Avoid cross-contamination

MIXING AND SETTING TIME:

No mixing. Apply for 10 seconds.

DIRECTIONS:

1. Place a couple of drops in a dappen dish.
2. Use a small applicator tip to dip into the dye.
3. Place the dye in the cavity preparation and let it set for about 10 seconds.
4. Rinse off the dye from the cavity preparation.
5. Burs and spoon excavators are used to remove the stained dentin.
6. This process is repeated until no caries remain.

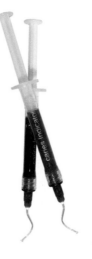

CARIES INDICATOR

MANUFACTURER:
Vista Dental Products

USE:
- Identification of carious dentin
- To preserve maximum amount of inner dentin while infected dentin is removed
- Assists in locating root canal orifices and calcified canals

COMPOSITION:
- Vista-Red   Glycol based with 1% acid red 52 solution
- Vista-Blue   Methylene blue solution 1%, water
- Vista-Green   Propylene glycol with FD&C green

PROPERTIES:
- Supplied in unit dose packages and prefilled syringes
- Must be rinsed off after reaction time of 10 seconds
- Do not use after expiration date

- Do not store at temperature above 77 degrees F (25 degrees C)
- Avoid exposure to sunlight

OSHA PRECAUTIONS:

- Eye and skin irritation possible
- Should not be ingested
- Product is flammable. Keep away from open flame.
- Avoid cross-contamination
- If ingested, may cause nausea and vomiting

MIXING AND SETTING TIME:

No mixing. Apply for 10 seconds.

DIRECTIONS:

1. Dispense a small amount in a dappen dish.
2. Use a small applicator tip to dip into the dye.
3. Place the dye in the cavity preparation and let it set for about 10 seconds.
4. Rinse off the dye from the cavity preparation.

5. Burs and spoon excavators are used to remove the stained dentin.
6. This process is repeated until no caries remain.

DESENSITIZERS

Desensitizers are agents used to reduce or eliminate the sensitivity of the teeth. Sensitivity may be caused by exposed dentin from abrasion; caries; abfraction associated with bruxism; leaking restoration, scaling, and root planing; and some restorative materials.

There are several categories of desensitizing agents including toothpastes, fluoride gel/varnish, inorganic salts, and resin agents. This chapter will cover the inorganic salts and resin agents. The toothpastes and fluorides will be covered in Chapter 8.

RELIEF GEL

MANUFACTURER:
Discus Dental

USE:
- Reduces sensitivity associated with thermal changes, tooth whitening, acid penetration, sweets, and/or direct contact
- Assists in preventing tooth decay by aiding in rebuilding enamel
- Improves luster of teeth

COMPOSITION:
- Potassium nitrate 5% and fluoride 0.240%

PROPERTIES:
- Comes in a gel and is mint flavored
- Also comes in a syringe for easy application

OSHA PRECAUTIONS:

- Eye and skin irritation possible
- Should not be ingested

MIXING AND SETTING TIMES:

There is no mixing required.

DIRECTIONS:

Patient may apply directly into whitening tray or apply with a soft toothbrush.

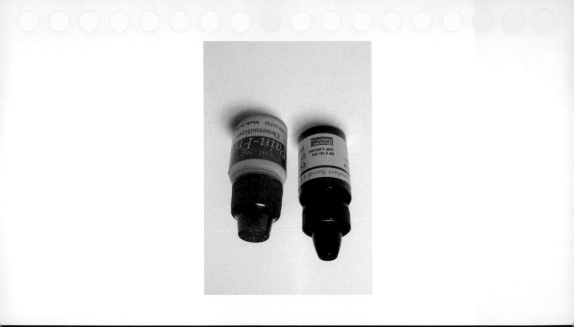

MANUFACTURER:
Heraeus Kulzer

USE:
- Prevents dentinal hypersensitivity
- Treats cervical sensitivity
- Prevents postoperative sensitivity
- Applied under amalgam restorations, with other bonding systems, under glass ionomers, under non-resin-bonded restorations, under resin-bonded veneers, inlays, onlays, and crowns
- Applied after root planing or periodontal treatment

COMPOSITION:
- 5% glutaraldehyde
- 35% HEMA-hydroxyethyl, methacrylate, pentanedial
- Water

PROPERTIES:
- Refrigerate if not used for long time
- Place pulp protection before placing Gluma if cavity preparation is close to pulp
- Drying the tooth before placement is not necessary; tooth can be moist.

OSHA PRECAUTIONS:
- Eye and skin irritation possible; if contact, rinse immediately
- Should not be ingested
- Product is flammable. Keep away from open flame.
- Avoid cross-contamination

MIXING AND SETTING TIME:
No mixing. Apply for 30 seconds.

DIRECTIONS:

1. Use a small sterile cotton pellet, applicator tip, or single dose applicator.
2. Apply material to the dentin of the tooth using a gentle but firm rubbing motion for 30 seconds.
3. Dry thoroughly but do not rinse.

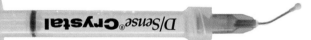

MANUFACTURER:
Centrix Dental

USE:
- Desensitizer and cavity liner
- Prevention of cervical erosion and gingival recession
- Applied under crowns and bridges, when standard cement is used
- Applied to exposed dentin, such as around the margins of a temporary crown
- Applied under restorations

COMPOSITION:
- Solution of potassium binoxalate and nitric acid in water
- Free of HEMA, glutaraldehyde, and other toxic chemicals

PROPERTIES:
- One-step, dual-action material
- Fast acting

- Long-lasting results
- Reacts with the dentin to precipitate microcrystals of calcium oxalate and potassium nitrate
- Occludes dentinal tubules with calcium oxalate and potassium nitrate
- Time saving and less waste
- Gentle on soft tissues

OSHA PRECAUTIONS:
- Eye and skin irritation possible
- If ingested. Give a solution of sodium bicarbonate or liquid antacid medication

MIXING AND SETTING TIME:
No mixing required. Setting (drying) time is 30 seconds using a gentle air spray or 2 minutes without the air spray.

DIRECTIONS:

1. Remove the cap from the syringe and securely attach a Sofneedle foam tip or dispense a few drops of liquid from the syringe into a dappen dish and use a small applicator.
2. To improve the comfort of the patient, warm the syringe to body temperature.
3. Check the flow of the material from the syringe on a paper pad and then pass the syringe to the dentist for placement.
4. The material is rubbed until the dentin is saturated for about 20 seconds.
5. After the material is placed, gently air-dry for 30 seconds or let air-dry for 2 minutes. The material has a frosty white precipitate.
6. Repeat if needed.

CAVITY LINERS AND LOW-STRENGTH BASES

Cavity liners and low-strength bases are used in the cavity preparation where there is little or no dentin to cover the pulp. They have a variety of uses including protecting and soothing the pulp. Some stimulate the formation of secondary dentin and some contain fluoride to strengthen the tooth.

Cavity liners and low-strength bases come in the following forms: powder/liquid, two paste systems, single tube, and syringes with disposable tips.

FUJI LINING LC

MANUFACTURER:
GC America, Inc.

USE:
- Permanent durable lining or low-strength base under all types of restorations

COMPOSITION:
- Silicate glass powder: containing calcium, aluminum, and fluoride (calcium fluoroaluminosilicate glass)
- Liquid: aqueous solution of polyacrylic acid

PROPERTIES:
- Light-cured material
- Releases fluoride
- Radiopaque material
- Biocompatible to reduce sensitivity

- Bonds mechanically and chemically to the tooth structure
- Also comes in paste form

OSHA PRECAUTIONS:
- Eye and skin irritation possible

MIXING AND SETTING TIME:
- Mixing time is 5 to 10 seconds for the first portion and 10 to 15 seconds for the second portion for a total not to exceed 20 seconds.
- Material is light-cured for approximately 30 seconds to set. (Time depends on strength of curing light.)
- Avoid long exposure to overhead light once the material is mixed.

DIRECTIONS:
1. Prepare materials. Powder and liquid, powder dispensing scoop specific to this product (or paste cartridge and dispenser), paper pad, 2 × 2 gauze, and placement instrument.
2. Tooth should be isolated with rubber dam or cotton rolls.

3. Rinse and dry the cavity preparation.
4. Dispense one level scoop of powder (scoop comes with kit).
   Replace the cap on the powder.
5. Divide the powder into two sections on the paper pad. Dispense one drop of liquid holding the bottle vertically upside down. Replace the cap on the liquid.
6. Incorporate the first portion into the liquid and mix for 5 to 10 seconds.
7. Then bring the second portion and mix the whole for 10 to 15 seconds. Total mixing time should not exceed 20 seconds.
8. Secure paste cartridge into the dispenser and dispense pastes onto the paper pad. Mix until smooth, uniform mix.
9. Apply the mix into the cavity preparation with a small applicator or suitable lining instrument.
10. Pass the instrument/applicator to the dentist and hold the paper pad and a gauze sponge close to the patient's chin for easy access during placement of the lining cement.
11. Once the material has been placed, light-cure for 30 seconds.

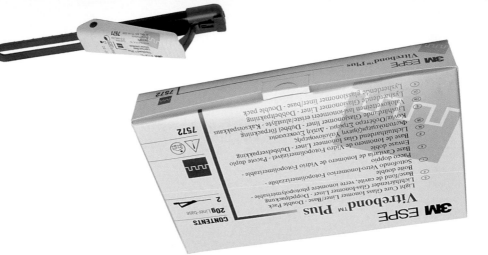

3M ESPE

Vitrebond™ Plus

CONTENTS

20g Liner-Base

7572

Vitrebond™ Plus
Light Cure Glass Ionomer Liner/Base - Double Pack
Lichthärtender Glas-Ionomer Liner - Doppelpackung
Base/fond double
Sottofondo doppio
Base Cavitária de Ionômero de Vidro Fotopolimerizável -
Envase doble
Base de Ionômero de Vidro Fotopolimerizável - Pacote dúplo
Lichthärtend Glas Ionomer Liner - Doppelverpackung
Φωτοπολυμεριζόμενη Υαλο Ιονομερική Βάση Επικάλυψης
Kovru/Обстерео Σπρυκ - Διπλό Εφλκτικαπλής
Lushärtande Glasionomeri Liner - Dubbel förpackning
Φωτοπολυμεριζόμενη γιασι-ιονομερική liner - Διπλό Σπρυκπαλς
Lushärdande Glasionomeri Liner/base - Dubbelpakking
Valokovettein lasi-ionomeeri Liner - Dobbelpakning
Lushärdende Glasionomeri Liner/base - Dobbelpakking
Lyshærdende glasionomer liner/base - Dobbeltpakking
Lysherdende glasionomer liner/base - Kaksoispakkaus

Vitrebond™ Plus

3M ESPE

7572

VITREBOND PLUS

MANUFACTURER:
3M ESPE

USE:
- Permanent liner/base
- Prevention of microleakage
- Aids in reducing the effects of polymerization shrinkage of the restorative materials
- Seals dentin to reduce postoperative sensitivity

COMPOSITION:
- Resin-modified glass ionomer-paste and liquid form

PROPERTIES:
- Strong bond to dentin
- Has the "clicker" dispensing system for easy use
- Less mess than powder/liquid systems
- Releases fluoride
- Good consistency and quick set

OSHA PRECAUTIONS:

- Eye and skin irritation possible

MIXING AND SETTING TIME:

Mix for 10 to 15 seconds. Light-cure for 20 seconds.

DIRECTIONS:

1. Prepare materials. Dual-barrel "clicker" dispensing gun, cement spatula, paper pad, 2 × 2 gauze, and placement instrument.
2. Tooth should be isolated with rubber dam or cotton rolls.
3. Rinse and dry the cavity preparation.
4. On a paper pad dispense a small amount of material from the dispenser until you hear the "click." This should give you equal amounts of the paste and liquid.
5. Gather the material with the cement spatula and mix for 10 to 15 seconds until the mix is uniform in color.
6. Pass the placement instrument to the dentist and hold the paper pad close to the patient's chin.
7. Once the material is in place, light-cure for 20 seconds.

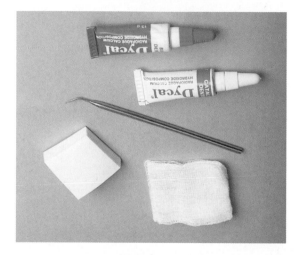

MANUFACTURER:
Dentsply Caulk

USE:
- A low-strength liner under any restoration, cements, and other base materials
- Applied with indirect or direct pulp capping procedures

COMPOSITION:
- Base-Zinc oxide, 1, 3 butylene glycol disalicylate, calcium phosphate, calcium tungstate, and iron oxide pigments
- Catalyst-Calcium hydroxide, N-ethyl-o/p-toluene sulfonamide, zinc oxide, titanium dioxide, zinc stearate, and iron oxide pigments (dentin shade only)

PROPERTIES:
- Rigid, self-setting material
- Radiopaque

- Has a therapeutic effect on the pulp
- Alkaline pH between 9 and 11, which stimulates the formation of secondary dentin when the material is in direct contact with the pulp
- Has some thermal insulating properties
- Minimal strength to support the forces of condensation

OSHA PRECAUTIONS:

- Some patients may be sensitive to calcium hydroxide cements.
- Eye contact—flush immediately with flowing water

MIXING AND SETTING TIME:

- Mix within 10 seconds
- Mixed material will set in 2 1/2 to 3 1/2 minutes
- Moisture and higher temperatures will decrease the working time and cause the material to set faster.

DIRECTIONS:

1. Prepare materials. Base and catalyst tubes, small paper pad, 2 × 2 gauze, and placement instrument (Dycal instrument or explorer).
2. Dispense equal amounts of the base and catalyst on the mixing pad provided.
3. Stir the two pastes together using the Dycal instrument or an explorer.
4. Mix for 10 seconds until a uniform color has been achieved.
5. Wipe the Dycal instrument off with a gauze sponge and pass to the dentist.
6. Hold the small paper pad with the mixed material close to the patient's chin for easy reach of the dentist.
7. Have a gauze sponge ready to remove any excess material during the application.

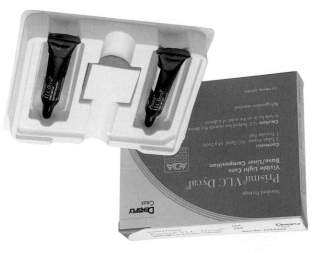

PRISMA VLC DYCAL

MANUFACTURER:
Dentsply Caulk

USE:
- A low-strength liner under any restoration, cements, and other base materials
- Applied with indirect or direct pulp capping procedures

COMPOSITION:
- Similar to two-paste calcium hydroxide with polymerizable monomers

PROPERTIES:
- Light-cured material
- Requires no mixing
- Must be refrigerated to prolong shelf life
- Radiopaque
- Material has a therapeutic effect on the pulp.

- Alkaline pH between 9 and 11, which stimulates the formation of secondary dentin when the material is in direct contact with the pulp
- Has some thermal insulating properties
- Minimal strength to support the forces of condensation
- Very low water solubility compared to two-paste calcium hydroxide

OSHA PRECAUTIONS:

- Some patients may be sensitive to calcium hydroxide cements.
- Eye contact—flush immediately with flowing water

MIXING AND SETTING TIME:

No mixing required. Setting time depends on curing light, but a minimum of 20 seconds is required.

DIRECTIONS:

1. Dispense Prisma VLC Dycal on a small paper pad and cover to avoid exposure to light. Allow the material to warm to room temperature.
2. Rinse and dry the cavity preparation.
3. Uncover the material, pass the Dycal instrument and hold the paper pad under the patient's chin for easy reach of the dentist.
4. Have a gauze sponge ready to remove any excess material during the application.
5. Prepare the curing unit and then cure the material for a minimum of 20 seconds with the light source within 2 mm of the material. If the curing unit is between 2 mm and 5 mm from the surface, cure the material for 30 seconds.

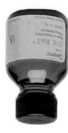

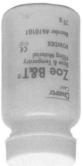

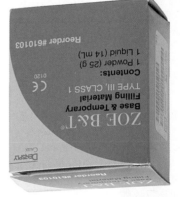

B & T BASE AND TEMPORARY CEMENT

MANUFACTURER:
Dentsply Caulk

USE:
- Intermediate base
- Temporary filling

COMPOSITION:
- Zinc oxide eugenol material (ZOE)
- Powder-zinc oxide, resin, zinc acetate, and an accelerator
- Liquid-eugenol and other oils such as clove oil

PROPERTIES:
- Very soluble in the mouth
- Low strength
- Has a neutral pH of 7, so this material is very compatible with the tooth
- Sedative effect on the tooth
- Does not require a protective base or liner

- Irritating to oral mucosa
- Has a strong odor
- May interfere with the polymerization process of composite materials

OSHA PRECAUTIONS:

- May irritate the eyes, skin, and oral mucosa tissues
- Inhalation—this material has a strong odor.

MIXING AND SETTING TIME:

- Mixing time—approximately 1 minute
- Setting time—2 1/2 to 3 1/2 minutes in the mouth

DIRECTIONS:

1. Prepare materials. Powder and liquid, paper pad, cement spatula, 2 × 2 gauze, and plastic filling instrument.
2. Tooth should be isolated with rubber dam or cotton rolls.
3. Rinse and dry the cavity preparation.

4. Place 2 or more drops of liquid on a mixing pad depending on the size of the cavity preparation.
5. Dispense sufficient powder and divide the powder into several small increments.
6. Bring the first portion of powder into the liquid and mix; continue to bring the rest of the powder into the mix for 1 minute. The mix should be a heavy nonsticky consistency that can be rolled into a ball.
7. Wipe off the spatula with gauze and pass a plastic filling instrument to the dentist.
8. During placement of the material, hold the paper pad with the mixed B & T near the patient's chin with gauze to remove any excess material.

CAVITY VARNISH

Cavity varnish is a material that is used as a protective barrier between the restoration and the prepared tooth. It seals the dentin tubules from irritating chemicals found in restorative materials and cements. Varnish sometimes comes with a solvent to thin the varnish when it becomes too thick for placement.

Cavity varnish is used in some cavity preparations but many dentists prefer to use a bonding agent that has multiple functions.

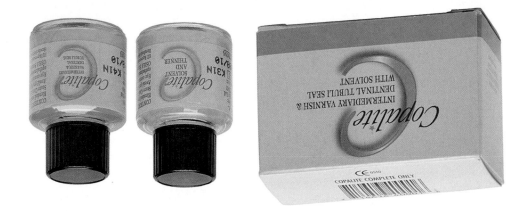

COPALITE

MANUFACTURER:
Cooley & Cooley, LTD

USE:
- Seals the dentin tubules
- Acts as a protective barrier

COMPOSITION:
- Natural resins
- Organic solvents (ether alcohol, acetone, or chloroform)

PROPERTIES:
- Has a strong odor
- Does not exhibit any strength
- Does not provide any thermal insulation
- Insoluble in the oral fluids
- Reduces microleakage
- Prevents penetration of acids from cements and restorative materials

- Non-acidic and non-irritating
- Solvent in the varnish will evaporate so it is important to keep the bottle tightly capped when not in use.

OSHA PRECAUTIONS:

- May irritate the eyes, skin, and oral mucosa tissues
- Inhalation—this material has a strong odor and may cause respiratory difficulties.
- Should not be ingested
- Product is flammable. Keep away from open flame.

MIXING AND SETTING TIME:

- No mixing required. Setting time: 5 to 10 seconds or just long enough for the layers to dry.

DIRECTIONS:

1. Clean and dry the cavity preparation.
2. Prepare two applicator brushes, cotton-tipped applicators, or small cotton pellets.

3. Remove the cap from the varnish and dip the applicators into the varnish until they are moistened.
4. Replace the cap on the varnish because of the strong odor and to prevent evaporation of solvent.
5. Dab off the excess varnish on a gauze.
6. One layer of varnish is placed on dentin in the cavity preparation and then allowed to dry.
7. Apply the second coat using the second applicator in the same manor and allow it to dry.

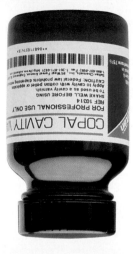

COPAL CAVITY VARNISH

MANUFACTURER:
Sultan Healthcare

USE:
- Protects dentin from acids released by filling materials
- Provides chemical and slight thermal protection while eliminating air pockets

COMPOSITION:
- Copal resins
- 75% dichloromethane

PROPERTIES:
- Needs no thinner
- Does not exhibit any strength
- Insoluble in the oral fluids
- Reduces microleakage

- Prevents penetration of acids from cements and restorative materials
- Non-acidic and non-irritating

OSHA PRECAUTIONS:

- May irritate the eyes, skin, and oral mucosa tissues
- Inhalation—this material has a strong odor.
- Should not be ingested
- Product is flammable. Keep away from open flame.

MIXING AND SETTING TIME:

- Comes in single bottle—no mixing required
- Setting time: 5 to 10 seconds just long enough for the layers to dry

DIRECTIONS:

1. Clean and dry the cavity preparation.
2. Prepare two applicator brushes, cotton-tipped applicators, or small cotton pellets.

3. Remove the cap from the varnish and dip the applicators into the varnish until they are moistened.
4. Replace the cap on the varnish because of the strong odor.
5. Dab off the excess varnish on a gauze.
6. One layer of varnish is placed on dentin in the cavity preparation and then allowed to dry.
7. Apply the second coat using the second applicator in the same manor and allow it to dry.

A core buildup is treatment performed on teeth that have very little crown structure left after the cavity preparation. The teeth are built up to support and provide retention for permanent restorations such as a porcelain crown.

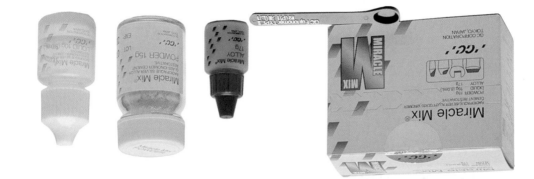

MIRACLE MIX

MANUFACTURER:
GC America, Inc.

USE:
- Crown and core buildup
- Block-outs and repairs

COMPOSITION:
- 100% fine silver alloy
- Glass ionomer cement
- Fluoride

PROPERTIES:
- Long-lasting
- Strong direct bond
- Color contrast with tooth structure
- Has high fluoride release to reduce secondary decay
- Easy to mix and place
- Won't stain or discolor surrounding teeth

- Shrinks and expands at the same rate as tooth structure
- Comes in a powder/liquid form and easy-to-use capsules

OSHA PRECAUTIONS:

- Eye and skin irritation is possible.
- Some patients are allergic to glass ionomer cements.

MIXING AND SETTING TIME:

- Powder/Liquid—Mixing time is 35 to 40 seconds.
- Capsules—Preparation time is 10 to 15 seconds.
- Setting time is 4 to 5 minutes for both forms.

DIRECTIONS:

Powder/Liquid

1. When using for the first time, pour the Miracle Mix alloy into the bottle of Miracle Mix powder and shake thoroughly.
2. Lightly tap the bottle for accurate dispensing of the powder.
3. Using the scoop that comes in the package, dispense 2 or 3 level scoops of powder on a paper pad.

4. Divide the powder into 2 equal parts.
5. Hold the liquid bottle vertically and squeeze to dispense 2 drops of liquid.
6. Mix the first portion with all the liquid for 15 to 20 seconds.
7. Incorporate the second portion and mix thoroughly for 20 seconds.
8. Mix will be thick and putty-like.
9. Transfer the cement to the dentist using a syringe or plastic filling instrument (PFI).

Capsule:
1. Tap the capsule on a flat surface to fluff the powder.
2. To activate the capsule, press the button on the bottom of the capsule.
3. Place the capsule in a high-speed amalgamator and triturate for 10 seconds.
4. Remove the capsule from the amalgamator and place it into the applier for delivery.

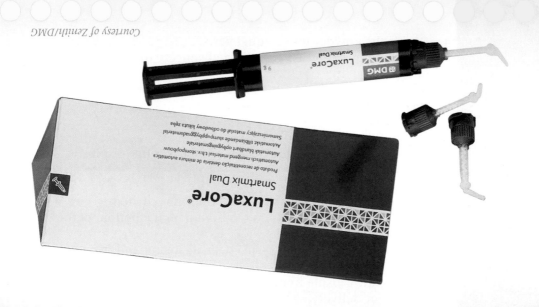
Courtesy of Zenith/DMG

LUXACORE DUAL SMARTMIX

MANUFACTURER:
Zenith/DMG

USE:
- One-step automix core buildup material

COMPOSITION:
- 72% filled composite resin material

PROPERTIES:
- Comes in a compact, self-contained syringe for a consistent mix every time
- No mixing, no air bubbles, and no wasted material
- Light-cured, self-cured, and dual-cured
- Strong resin material
- Releases fluoride to protect against secondary caries
- Syringe delivery for easy use and less chance of cross-contamination

- Comes in three colors-natural A3 for optimal esthetics, blue for contrast with the tooth, and white for perfect balance of contrast and esthetics
- Increased work time
- Radiopaque on radiographs
- Composite viscosity to prevent material from slumping before cured

OSHA PRECAUTIONS:
- May cause skin and eye irritation
- Prolonged exposure may cause respiratory irritation.
- If ingested, rinse mouth out with water and contact a physician.

MIXING AND SETTING TIME:
- No mixing required.
- Setting Time: Light-cure according to size of buildup—20 to 40 seconds

DIRECTIONS:

1. The tooth is prepared and then rinsed and dried.
2. Prepare the Smartmix handheld double-barreled syringe by removing the storage cap.
3. Place on small core tip or an intraoral tip.
4. Dispense a small amount of material on a paper pad or gauze to ensure material is mixed.
5. Pass the syringe to the dentist and have a PFI ready.
6. Once the material is placed, pass the curing light or light-cure the material when the dentist indicates he/she is ready. Depending on the depth of the core material, the curing time will vary.

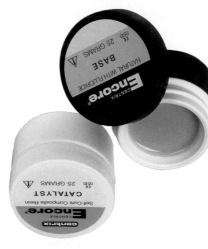

ENCORE CORE PASTE

MANUFACTURER:
Centrix Dental

USE:
- Core buildup material

COMPOSITION:
- Self-cured composite material
- Two-paste system that is used with a syringe for placement

PROPERTIES:
- High compressive strength
- Cuts like dentin to reduce ditching
- Comes with and without fluoride
- Radiopaque
- Comes in two shades: natural and white
- No slumping, therefore a matrix is not needed

OSHA PRECAUTIONS:

- May be irritating to the skin and eyes
- Should not be ingested
- Inhalation irritation—keep area well ventilated

MIXING AND SETTING TIME:

- Mixing time is 10 to 15 seconds. Working time is 2 1/2 minutes.
- Setting time is 4 to 5 minutes.

DIRECTIONS:

1. Prepare the tooth and apply the bonding agents.
2. Using one end of the spatula, take a small portion of the base.
3. Using the other end of the spatula, take a small and equal portion of the catalyst. Be sure not to cross-contaminate the two jars of material.
4. Mix the two materials together to a uniform mix. Working time at this point is 2 1/2 minutes.

5. Place the material into the Centrix C-R syringe tube. Fill half full.
6. Place the plug in the end of the tube.
7. Place the syringe tube into the syringe barrel and dispense a small amount of material to test the flow.
8. Pass the syringe to the dentist for placement.

BONDING AGENTS

Bonding agents are used to attach restorative materials to the enamel or dentin of the tooth. There are many varieties of materials; they are self-curing, light-cured, or dual-cured. Most often they require a conditioning or etching prior to placement. Some are unidose meaning the etchant and the bonding agent are placed at the same time, whereas others require the etchant to be placed as a separate step.

ADPER PROMPT L-POP SELF-ETCH ADHESIVE

MANUFACTURER:
3M ESPE

USE:
- Adhesive for direct restorative procedures

COMPOSITION:
- Low-viscosity composite resin
- Di–hema phosphate
- Bisphone a diglycidyl ether dimethacrylate
- Ethyl 4 dimethyl aminobenzoate
- Dl camphoquinone

PROPERTIES:
- Improved properties for better bonding
- Higher viscosity for even application
- Easy application
- Etches, primes, and bonds in one step
- Aggressive etchant

- Reduces postoperative sensitivity
- Easy-to-use technique
- Comes in a unit-dose or vial delivery system (Adper Prompt Self-Etch Adhesive 3M ESPE)

OSHA PRECAUTIONS:

- May be irritating to the skin and eyes
- Should not be ingested
- No inhalation irritation

MIXING AND SETTING TIME:

- Mixing time is less than 5 seconds. (Refer to the directions.)
- Setting time is 10 seconds to light-cure.

DIRECTIONS:

1. Tooth is rinsed and lightly dried.
2. Press on the red chamber to move the contents into the yellow chamber.
3. Fold the red chamber over the yellow chamber.

4. The yellow chamber will pop up to indicate the material has flowed into this area.
5. Press again and the material will flow into the next chamber.
6. With the applicator, mix and churn the material to complete the mix.
7. Apply the material to the tooth by rubbing for 15 seconds.
8. Reapply until the surface is smooth and glossy.
9. The adhesive will appear a dull yellow.
10. Light-cure for 10 seconds.

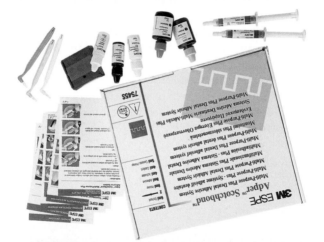

Courtesy of 3M ESPE

SCOTCHBOND MULTI-PURPOSE PLUS DENTAL ADHESIVE-ADPER 3M ESPE

MANUFACTURER:
3M ESPE

USE:
- Dual-curing adhesive for bonding fresh amalgams, self-cured composites, and porcelains
- Bonding system for indirect restoration including crowns, inlays, and onlays

COMPOSITION:
- Primer contains HEMA
- Catalyst contains HEMA and bis–GMA (low-viscosity composite resin)

PROPERTIES:
- Excellent bond strength to a variety of surfaces
- Fast and easy application
- Reduces microleakage and postoperative sensitivity

OSHA PRECAUTIONS:

- May be irritating to the skin and eyes
- Should not be ingested
- No inhalation irritation

MIXING AND SETTING TIME:

- There is no mixing required.
- Material is light-cured for 10 seconds.

DIRECTIONS:

1. Material works best if the tooth is isolated with a rubber dam.
2. Tooth is prepared, rinsed, and dried.
3. The etchant is applied to the enamel and dentin—wait 15 seconds.
4. Rinse thoroughly and then gently air-dry, leaving the tooth moist.
5. Apply Scotchbond Multi-Purpose Adhesive primer to the enamel and dentin with an applicator brush.

6. Gently dry for 5 seconds—the surface should appear shiny.
7. Apply Scotchbond Multi-Purpose Adhesive to the enamel and dentin with an applicator brush.
8. Light-cure for 10 seconds.

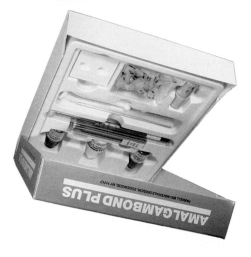
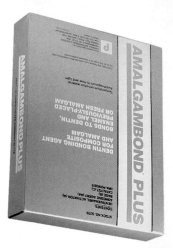

AMALGAMBOND PLUS ADHESIVE SYSTEM

MANUFACTURER:
Parkell, Inc.

USE:
- Bonding system for amalgams and composites to dentin, enamel, and existing amalgams
- Pulp capping

COMPOSITION:
- Low-viscosity composite resin

PROPERTIES:
- Provides a high-power bond
- Reduces the needs for pins
- Reduces sensitivity
- No need to place varnish or liners
- Reduces microleakage

OSHA PRECAUTIONS:

- May be irritating to the skin and eyes
- Should not be ingested
- May be inhalation irritation

MIXING AND SETTING TIME:

- Mix the base and catalyst for 3 to 5 seconds.
- Allow the dentin activator to dry for 30 seconds.
- Allow the adhesive agent to dry for 30 seconds.
- Allow the base and catalyst to dry before placing composite material for 60 seconds.

DIRECTIONS:

1. Pumice the tooth, then rinse and dry completely.
2. Dispense 1 or 2 drops of dentin activator into the mixing well.
3. Brush the activator on the dentin for 10 seconds—to etch the enamel leave on for 30 seconds.
4. Wash and dry the area.
5. Dispense 1 or 2 drops of adhesive agent into a clean mixing well.

6. Brush a thin layer of the adhesive onto the activated dentin surface.
7. Air-dry the surface to achieve an even, thin layer of coverage.
8. Leave for 30 seconds.
9. Dispense 2 drops of base and 1 drop of catalyst into a clean mixing well.
10. Mix thoroughly for 3 to 5 seconds.
11. Brush a thin, even layer onto the cavity preparation.
12. Place the amalgam immediately before the adhesive dries. If placing a composite, allow the adhesive to dry about 60 seconds before placing the composite.

OPTIBOND SOLO PLUS SYSTEM

MANUFACTURER:
Kerr Corporation

USE:
- Adhesive for direct and indirect bonding
- Different bonding applications—either unidose or self-curing bottle delivery
- Caries protection
- Pulp capping

COMPOSITION:
- Micron-filled composite resin with ethanol

PROPERTIES:
- High bond strength to a variety of surfaces
- Protects against sensitivity
- Prevents microleakage

- Caries protection
- Fluoride release
- Reduces shrinkage
- No need for liners or varnish

OSHA PRECAUTIONS:
- May be irritating to the skin and eyes
- Should not be ingested
- Inhalation irritation may occur

MIXING AND SETTING TIME:
- If mixing is required, mix for 3 seconds.
- Material is light-cured for 20 seconds.

DIRECTIONS:
OptiBond Solo in Unidose (capsule or rocket) delivery
1. Etch the enamel and dentin for 15 seconds.
2. Rinse thoroughly and lightly air-dry.

3. Grip the unidose capsule at the wings and twist each side in opposite directions.
4. Discard the larger end.
5. Place one drop of OptiBond Solo Plus Activator into open end of the capsule.
6. Dip an applicator tip into the opening and mix for 3 seconds.
7. Apply the OptiBond Solo Plus for 15 seconds.
8. Light-cure fore 20 seconds.

OptiBond Solo Plus in Bottles

1. Etch the enamel and dentin for 15 seconds.
2. Rinse thoroughly and lightly air-dry.
3. Place one drop of OptiBond Solo Plus and one drop of OptiBond Solo Plus Activator into the mixing well and mix for 3 seconds.
4. Apply for 15 seconds.
5. Air-dry gently for 3 seconds.

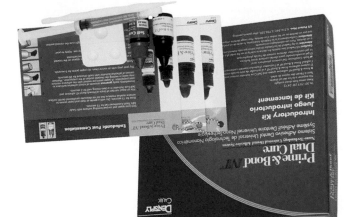

PRIME & BOND NT DUAL CURE NANO-TECHNOLOGY
DENTAL ADHESIVE

MANUFACTURER:
Dentsply Caulk

USE:
- Universal self-priming dental adhesive
- Direct composites and compomers
- Veneers
- Indirect restorations, inlay, onlays, crowns, and bridges
- Repairs on composites, ceramics, and amalgams
- Endodontic post-cementation
- Adhesive bonding of direct amalgam bonding

COMPOSITION:
- Dimethacrylate resin and acetone
- Highly filled nano-filled composite

PROPERTIES:
- Superior bond
- Protection against microleakage

- Better surface coverage and penetration into dentin
- High bond strength

OSHA PRECAUTIONS:

- May be irritating to the skin and eyes
- Should not be ingested
- Inhalation irritation may occur

MIXING AND SETTING TIME:

- No mixing is required.
- Light-cure to set material

DIRECTIONS:

1. Rinse and dry the cavity preparation or if no cavity preparation is needed. Clean with a rubber cup and pumice or prophy paste and then rinse with water and air-dry.
2. Apply calcium hydroxide liner if necessary.
3. Condition/etch the tooth if required for 10 to 15 seconds and then rinse.

4. Gently air-dry-tooth can still be moist.
5. Dispense Prime and Bond NT adhesive directly on an applicator brush or dispense 2 or 3 drops into a dispensing well. Replace the cap immediately.
6. Apply the adhesive on the tooth generously so the surface is wet. Additional application may be needed to keep the surface wet for 20 seconds.
7. Gently air-dry for 5 seconds; the surface should be glossy. If not, repeat the application of the adhesive.
8. Light-cure for 10 seconds and then place the restoration.

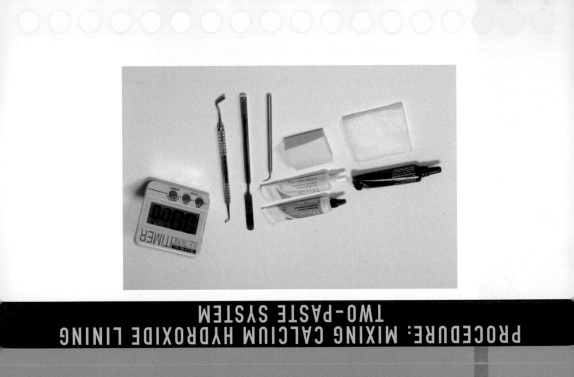

PROCEDURE: MIXING CALCIUM HYDROXIDE LINING
TWO-PASTE SYSTEM

This procedure is performed by the dental assistant at chairside after the dentist has completed the cavity preparation.

EQUIPMENT AND SUPPLIES:

- Calcium hydroxide two-paste system
- Small paper pad
- Small ball-ended instrument (often called the Dycal instrument) or an explorer
- 2 × 2 gauze sponge
- PPE worn by the dental assistant

DIRECTIONS:

1. After the dentist has completed the tooth preparation and the dental assistant has rinsed and dried the tooth, the liner is prepared to be placed.
2. Dispense small and equal amounts of both the catalyst and base onto the paper pad. The amount is determined by the size of the tooth and the preparation.
3. Wipe off the ends of the tubes and replace the caps.

4. Mix the two materials together using a circular motion.
5. Mix until the materials are a uniform color within the 10 to 15 second mixing time.
6. Wipe the excess material from the mixing instrument.
7. The dental assistant holds the paper pad, 2×2 gauze, and placement instrument ready to pass to the dentist.
8. Pass the instrument to the dentist and hold the paper pad close to the patient's chin.
9. Wipe off the instrument with the gauze for the dentist between applications.
10. Receive the instrument, wipe it off, tear and fold the top page of the paper pad, and dispose of it.

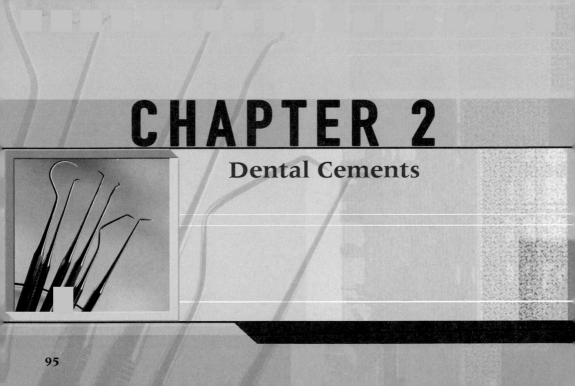

CHAPTER 2

Dental Cements

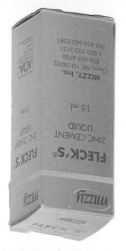
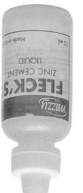
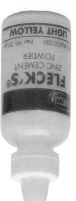
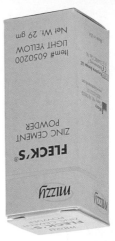

ZINC PHOSPHATE CEMENT—FLECK'S CEMENT

MANUFACTURER:

Mizzy, Inc.

USE:

- Permanent cement for indirect restorations including inlays, onlays, crowns, and bridges
- Orthodontic cement
- High-strength base

COMPOSITION:

- Powder—zinc oxide, magnesium oxide, and pigments
- Liquid—phosphoric acid and water

PROPERTIES:

- High strength
- May be irritating to the pulp, so a liner is used first
- Has an exothermic reaction when mixed
- Specific guidelines for mixing to minimize the temperature rise and slow the reaction process and improve the strength

OSHA PRECAUTIONS:

- Eye and skin irritation possible
- Should not be ingested
- Avoid cross-contamination

MIXING AND SETTING TIME:

- Mixing time is 2 minutes.
- Working time is 3 1/2 minutes.
- Setting time is 2 to 8 minutes.

DIRECTIONS:

1. Obtain a clean, cool, dry glass slab and flexible cement spatula.
2. Fluff the powder and dispense appropriate amount for cementation.
3. Divide the powder in half, then divide into fourths, then divide one of the fourths into two eighths, and then one of the eighths into two sixteenths.
4. Dispense the liquid (6 to 12 drops) holding the dropper vertical to the glass slab.

5. Incorporate one-sixteenth portion of powder into the liquid and mix for 15 seconds. Repeat by adding the second sixteenth and mix for 15 seconds.
6. Add the eighth portion and mix the material using three quarters of the glass slab for 15 seconds.
7. Add one of the quarters and spatulate for 20 seconds; follow by a second quarter, which is also spatulated for 20 seconds.
8. Add enough of the last quarter of powder to achieve the consistency the dentist requires. Mix should be completed in 2 minutes.
9. For cementation, the consistency is fluid and should follow the spatula up about an inch from the glass slab.
10. Using the PFI, prepare to pass the cement to the dentist. Have the gauze ready to remove any excess cement from the spatula.
11. Clean the glass slab and spatula immediately.
12. For the base consistency, add more powder to the liquid until you reach a putty-like consistency and the cement can be rolled into a ball.

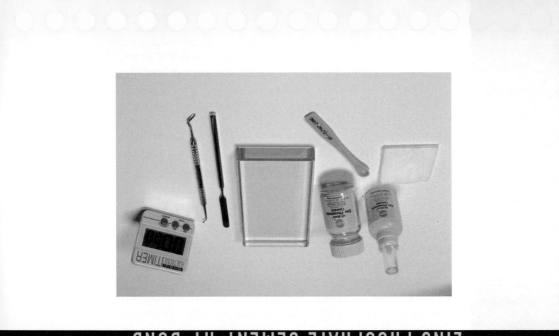

MANUFACTURER:

Shofu Dental Corporation

USE:

- Permanent cement to bond metal crowns, bridges, inlays, and onlays
- Bonds orthodontic appliances

COMPOSITION:

- Powder—zinc oxide, magnesium oxide, and pigments
- Liquid—phosphoric acid and water

PROPERTIES:

- High compressive strength
- Contains tannin fluoride
- Radiopaque
- May be irritating to the pulp

OSHA PRECAUTIONS:

- Eye and skin irritation possible
- Should not be ingested
- Avoid cross-contamination

MIXING AND SETTING TIME:

- Mixing time is within 60 seconds.
- Working time is 3 1/2 minutes.
- Setting time is 6 1/2 minutes from the end of the mix.

DIRECTIONS:

1. Obtain a clean, cool, dry glass slab and flexible cement spatula.
2. Fluff the powder and use the Shofu spoon to dispense one scoop of powder. Use the straight edge of the semicircular hole in the stopper to level the powder.
3. Divide the powder into three equal portions.
4. Dispense four drops of liquid onto the glass slab.
5. Bring in the first portion and mix with short, quick strokes until the mix is homogeneous.

6. Repeat with the next two portions until all of the powder is incorporated into a smooth homogeneous mix.
7. Prepare to pass the cement to the dentist, having the PFI and a gauze pad ready.

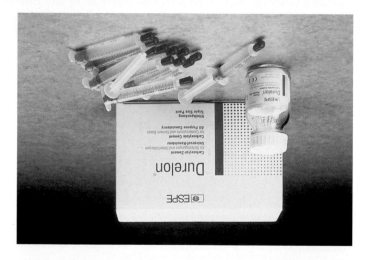

POLYCARBOXYLATE CEMENT–DURELON

MANUFACTURER:
3M ESPE

USE:
- Permanent cement for crowns, bridges, inlays, and onlays
- Orthodontic cementation
- High-strength base

COMPOSITION:
- Powder is zinc oxide with small amounts of magnesium oxide.
- Stannous fluoride
- Liquid is polyacrylic acid copolymer in water.
- Liquid comes in a squeeze bottle or calibrated syringe.

PROPERTIES:
- High strength
- Does not exhibit exothermic heat
- Bonds chemically to the tooth structure and mechanically to the restoration

- More viscous
- Less irritating
- Has a shelf life and should be discarded if the liquid discolors and becomes thick

OSHA PRECAUTIONS:

- Eye and skin irritation possible
- Should not be ingested
- Avoid cross-contamination

MIXING AND SETTING TIME:

- Mixing time is a minimum of 30 seconds.
- Working time is 2 minutes.
- Setting time is 5 to 10 minutes.

DIRECTIONS:

Using powder and squeeze bottle

1. Gather the paper pad, cement spatula, powder, dosing rod, liquid, and gauze.

2. Fluff the powder and then, using the dosing rod, measure and dispense one scoop of powder on the paper pad. Press the dosing rod into the powder and then, using the spatula, remove excess powder before placing on the paper pad.
3. Dispense the liquid by holding the squeeze bottle vertical and drop 2 drops onto the paper pad next to the powder.
4. Mix all the powder into the liquid in one move and mix until a uniform, homogeneous consistency is attained, approximately 30 seconds.
5. Gather the cement and prepare to pass to the dentist. Use wet gauze to remove excess material before it sets on the spatula and placement instrument.

Using powder and calibrated syringe

1. Prepare the powder as described above.
2. Dispense the liquid from the syringe using the calibrations. For one scoop of powder use two scale units of liquid.
3. Mix all the powder into the liquid in one move until a uniform, homogeneous consistency is attained, approximately 30 seconds.

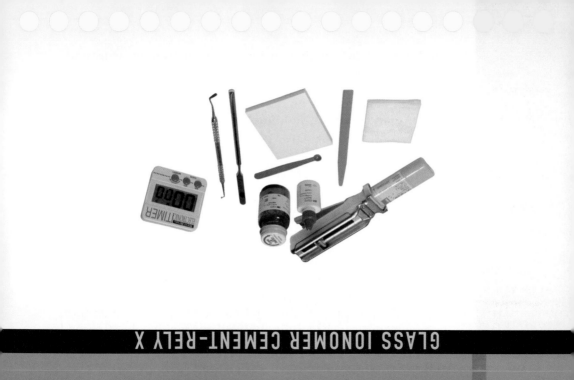

MANUFACTURER:
3M ESPE

USE:
- Cementing porcelain fused to metal crowns and bridges, amalgam composite, or glass ionomer core buildups
- Metal inlays, onlays, and crowns
- Prefabricated and cast post cementation
- Cementation of orthodontic appliances

COMPOSITION:
- Powder is a radiopaque fluoroaluminosilicate glass.
- Liquid is an aqueous solution of modified polyalkenoic acid.

PROPERTIES:
- High strength
- Chemically adheres to tooth structure and restoration
- Releases fluoride
- Low solubility

- Low viscosity, non-stringy, slump-resistant mix
- Non-irritating qualities
- Easy to mix and clean up

OSHA PRECAUTIONS:

- Eye and skin irritation possible
- Should not be ingested
- May cause mild respiratory irritation
- Contains HEMA, which is a known allergen

MIXING AND SETTING TIME:

- Mixing time is 30 seconds.
- Working time is 2 1/2 minutes from the start of the mix at room temperature.
- Setting time is within 10 minutes.

DIRECTIONS:

Comes in a powder/liquid system and a clicker dispenser system

Powder/Liquid System

1. Gather a paper pad, cement spatula, and gauze.
2. Keep the caps on the powder and liquid when not in use.
3. Fluff the powder. Using the specific scoop that is supplied with Rely X, dispense 3 scoops of powder on the paper pad. Three scoops of powder and 3 drops of liquid is adequate to seat one typical crown. Use an equal number of powder scoops and liquid drops.
4. Holding the squeeze bottle vertical, dispense 3 uniform-sized drops.
5. Bring all the powder into the liquid and mix in a small area to minimize water evaporation and maximize working time. Complete the mix in 30 seconds.
6. The mix should be smooth and uniform.
7. Prepare to pass the cement to the dentist. Use a gauze to wipe the excess from the spatula and PFI.

Clicker Dispenser System

1. Dispense one portion to ensure that the dispenser is working correctly.
2. Dispose of the test material and on new paper squeeze the dispenser until you hear a clicking, continue to dispense one to three clicks depending on the restoration(s) to be cemented.
3. Mix the material into a homogeneous mix within 30 seconds. It is then ready for cementation.

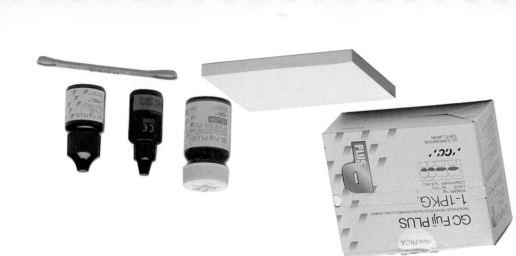

FUJI-GLASS IONOMER LUTING CEMENT

MANUFACTURER:
GC America

USE:
- For final cementation of crown and bridge restorations
- Metal inlays, onlays, posts
- Orthodontic appliances

COMPOSITION:
- Powder is a radiopaque fluoroaluminosilicate glass.
- Liquid is polyacrylic acid and water.

PROPERTIES:
- Strong direct bond
- Marginal integrity for long-term restorations
- Minimizes microleakage
- Releases fluoride
- Does not require a dry field

- Low film thickness and low solubility
- Easy to mix and clean up

OSHA PRECAUTIONS:

- Eye and skin irritation possible
- Should not be ingested
- May cause mild respiratory irritation

MIXING AND SETTING TIME:

- Mixing time is 20 to 30 seconds depending on the size of the mix.
- Setting time is approximately 5 minutes.

DIRECTIONS:

Powder/Liquid System

1. Gather the paper pad, cement spatula, and gauze.
2. Keep the caps on the powder and liquid when not in use.

3. Fluff the powder. Using the specific scoop that is supplied with Fuji, dispense 1 scoop of powder on the paper pad. Divide the powder into two equal parts.
4. Holding the squeeze bottle vertical, dispense 2 uniform-sized drops.
5. Mix the first portion for 10 to 15 seconds with the liquid. Add the second portion and mix for 15 to 20 seconds.
6. Mix in a small area to minimize water evaporation and maximize working time. Complete the mix in 20 to 30 seconds.
7. The mix should be smooth and uniform.
8. Prepare to pass the cement to the dentist. Use a gauze to wipe the excess from the spatula and PFI.

Premeasured Capsules
1. Tap the capsule on a flat surface to fluff the powder.
2. Depress the button on the bottom of the capsule to activate.
3. Place the capsule in a high-speed amalgamator and triturate for 10 seconds.
4. Place in designated dispenser. It is ready to use.

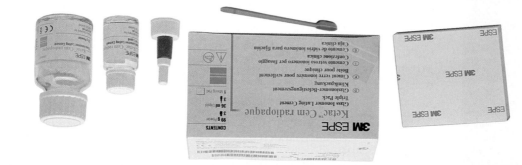

KETAC-CEM RADIOPAQUE, KETAC-CEM APLICAP, AND KETAC-CEM MAXICAP

MANUFACTURER:

3M ESPE

USE:

- All of these materials are used for permanent cementation of inlays, crowns, bridges, and orthodontic bands/brackets.

COMPOSITION:

- Powder is a calcium-aluminum-fluorosilicate glass.
- Liquid is polyacrylic acid and water.

PROPERTIES:

- High compressive strength
- Adheres chemically to tooth structure
- Very low solubility
- Adheres to slightly moist tooth structure
- Minimal film thickness
- Releases fluoride ions to tooth structure
- Comes in various forms for easy use and cleanup
- Non-irritating to the pulp

OSHA PRECAUTIONS:

- Eye and skin irritation possible
- Should not be ingested
- May cause mild respiratory irritation

MIXING AND SETTING TIME:

- Powder/Liquid mix—Mixing time is 60 seconds.
- Aplicap and MAXICAP—10 seconds
- Setting time for all is 7 minutes.

DIRECTIONS:

Powder/Liquid Mix

1. Gather a paper pad, cement spatula, and gauze.
2. Keep the caps on the powder and liquid when not in use.
3. Fluff the powder. Using the specific scoop that is supplied with Ketac-Cem, dispense 1 scoop of powder on the paper pad.
4. Holding the squeeze bottle vertical, dispense 2 uniform-sized drops.

5. Mix the powder into the liquid in one portion. Mix for 60 seconds until the mix is smooth and has a glossy appearance. When the surface becomes dull, the setting reaction has started and the mix should be discarded.
6. Prepare to pass the cement to the dentist. Use a gauze to wipe the excess from the spatula and PFI.

Aplicap and MAXICAP

1. Both of these systems are prepared in the same manner; the difference is in the amount of cement. The MAXICAP capsules contain a larger mix than the Aplicaps.
2. Shake the capsule to fluff the powder and then place in the designated activator to release the liquid into the powder in the capsule.
3. Place the capsule in the amalgamator and triturate for 10 seconds.
4. Remove the capsule from the amalgamator and place in the designated applier.
5. Materials are ready to dispense at this point.

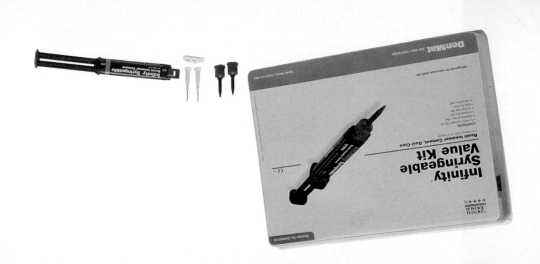

MANUFACTURER:
Den-Mat Corporation

USE:
- All-purpose cement for porcelain-metal, all ceramic, resin inlays, onlays, crowns, and bridges
- Maryland bridge cementation
- Endodontic post and core cementations
- Orthodontic band and bracket cementation

COMPOSITION:
- Resin-based fluoro-alumina silica glass

PROPERTIES:
- Self-adhesive and self-etching
- High-strength and long-lasting
- No bonding agent required in most cases
- Automixing syringe system
- Dual-curing

- Easy placement and cleanup
- Reduces postoperative sensitivity
- Prevents microleakage
- Stress-resistant margins—fracture resistant
- Low film thickness

OSHA PRECAUTIONS:

- Eye and skin irritation possible
- Should not be ingested
- May cause mild respiratory irritation

MIXING AND SETTING TIME:

- Automix dispenser—no mix is required.
- Margins can be light-cured for easy removal of excess cement.
- Setting time is approximately 5 minutes.

DIRECTIONS:

1. Clean the tooth surface thoroughly.
2. Roughen a composite or metal surface with a micro-etcher or by sandblasting before placing the cement.
3. Remove the cap from the syringe. Dispense a small amount of Infinity on a mixing pad. Wipe the end of the syringe tips with a tissue.
4. Align the automixing tip with the notch in the syringe and then turn the tip clockwise until it stops turning.
5. Hand the syringe to the dentist for dispensing on the restoration and the tooth.
6. When finished, remove the automixing tip and place the cap back on the syringe.
7. Excess cement is removed and then the patient should bite on the restoration for another 5 minutes.

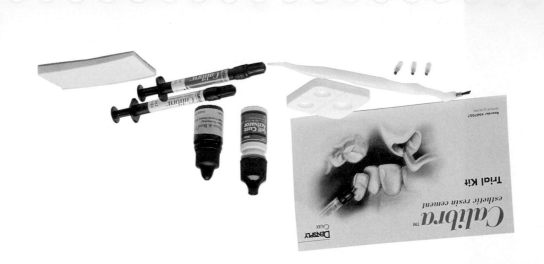

MANUFACTURER:
Dentsply Caulk

USE:
- Resin cement for all indirect esthetic restorations including: ceramic, porcelain composite inlays/onlays, veneers, and crowns
- Cement for all metal crowns, bridges, and inlays/onlays
- Cement for PFM (porcelain fused to metal crowns and bridges)
- Cement for prefabricated and cast posts
- Adhesive cement for resin-bonded Maryland bridges

COMPOSITION:
- Barium boron fluoro alumino silicate glass, Bis-GMA, polymerizable dimethacrylic resin, hydrophobic amorphous silica, Benzoyl peroxide
- Shades: inorganic iron oxides and titanium dioxide

PROPERTIES:

- High bond strength
- Virtually no sensitivity
- Long-term shade stability
- Variety of shades for excellent esthetics
- Low film thickness
- Light-cured and dual-cured
- Long-term retention
- Easy to handle and clean up
- Can be mixed to a variety of viscosities
- Do not use after expiration date

OSHA PRECAUTIONS:

- May cause irritation to the eyes and skin
- Do not breathe vapor
- Keep away from sources of ignition

MIXING AND SETTING TIME:

- Mixing time is 20 to 30 seconds.

- Working time is 2 minutes 30 seconds.
- Light-cured setting time is 20 seconds in each direction. Dual-cure is 6 minutes from the beginning of the mix.

DIRECTIONS:

1. Remove all temporary material from the tooth and polish with a rubber cup and pumice or non-fluoride cleaning paste. Wash thoroughly and lightly air-dry.
2. The inside of the restoration is microetched and after the try-in is completed, it is cleaned to remove all debris. Rinse in an ultrasonic cleaner, then apply Caulks Tooth Conditioner (etchant) for 30 seconds, and then rinse the restoration thoroughly with water for 20 seconds. Air-dry.
3. Keep the area isolated. Apply Calibra Silane Coupling Agent with the syringe to etch the surface and allow to dry.
4. The tooth is prepared in the same maner as the restoration. First, rinse the preparation and then dry. Apply the Tooth Conditioner for at least 15 seconds and then rinse for 10 seconds and then blot-dry with a moist cotton pellet. Do not rub the surfaces.

5. Dispense 1 to 2 drops of Prime & Bond NT into a mixing well; add an equal number of drops of the Self-Cure Activator. Mix and then apply with a disposable brush (see Chapter 1 Preliminary Restorative Dental Material, under Bonding Agents) to the tooth for 20 seconds and then light-cure. Apply Prime & Bond NT to the restoration for 10 seconds and then air-dry for 5 seconds.

6. On a paper pad, dispense the selected shade of Calibra's base and then an equal portion of the catalyst. Mix for 20 to 30 seconds.

7. After the cement is placed and the restoration is seated, light-cure for 20 seconds from each direction—buccal, lingual, and occlusal.

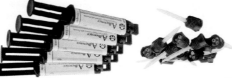
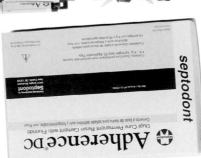

RESIN CEMENT–ADHERENCE ® DC

MANUFACTURER:

Septodont Inc.

USE:

- Final cementation of implant prostheses, bridges, crowns, inlay/onlays, Maryland bridges, and veneers. Including ceramic, metal, and metal to metal
- Cement for pins and posts

COMPOSITION:

- Base: Quartz and silica
- Catalyst: Resin: Bis-GMA, polyethyleneglycal dimethacrylate, benzoyl peroxide

PROPERTIES:

- Strong bonding
- Low film thickness
- Radiopaque
- Resistance to fracture

- Low solubility
- Not acidic

OSHA PRECAUTIONS:

- May cause irritation to the eyes and skin
- Do not breathe vapor
- Avoid elevated temperatures

MIXING AND SETTING TIME:

- Mixing time is 20 seconds.
- No mixing time is required for automix.
- Initial set is 1 1/2 minutes and final set is 3 1/2 minutes.

DIRECTIONS:

1. As with the other resin cements, the tooth and the restoration need to be prepared before mixing. Refer to Calibra for the steps of preparation.
2. Adherence DC does require a bonding system to be placed first. (Refer to Chapter 1, Bonding Agents.)

3. When ready, mix an equal amount of Adherence DC base and catalyst for 20 seconds or dispense on a paper pad or directly on permanent restoration with automix material.
4. Pass to the dentist and have the PFI ready or the injection syringe system.
5. The cement is placed on the tooth and in the restoration. The restoration is seated and held in place for 1 1/2 minutes.
6. Remove excess cement at this point.

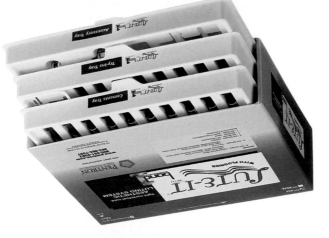

RESIN CEMENT-LUTE-IT

MANUFACTURER:
Pentron Clinical Technologies, LLC

USE:
- Cementing all composite and all ceramic indirect restorations including: veneers, inlays/onlays, crowns
- For intraoral porcelain repairs

COMPOSITION:
- BIS-GMA, UDMA, HDDMA, barium-borosilicate glass filler, inorganic fluoride, silica, Silane, photo initiator, amine, and inorganic pigments, benzoyl peroxide, and stabilizers

PROPERTIES:
- Light-cured resin with dual-cure option
- Low cost
- Versatile shading with three levels of opacity. Shades are more natural in appearance.
- Unique formula provides excellent long-term marginal integrity.

- Radiopaque
- Releases fluoride

OSHA PRECAUTIONS:

- Avoid contact on skin and in eyes.
- Some people may be allergic to the methacrylate resin.
- Avoid swallowing.

MIXING AND SETTING TIME:

- Mixing time is approximately 30 seconds.
- Dual-curing cement is 3 1/2 minutes working time.
- Setting time is about 4 minutes.

DIRECTIONS:

1. Choose the shade, reviewing the information concerning the actions of Lute-It cement.
2. Tooth Preparation—Etch the tooth for 20 seconds and rinse thoroughly.
3. A critical step is to keep the tooth moist. Either blot the tooth gently or use the air for 1 to 2 seconds.

4. Place two coats of Bond 1-Primer/Adhesive to the tooth for 10 seconds.
5. A critical step is to remove the solvent by gently using the air for at least 10 seconds.
6. Light-cure for 10 seconds.
7. Restoration Preparation—Apply Lute-It Silane to the inside of the restoration that has been etched, micro-etched, or sandblasted. Leave Silane on for 1 minute and then dry.
8. Apply one coat of Bond 1-Primer/Adhesive to the inside of the restoration. Remove the solvent by gently using the air for at least 10 seconds. Do not light-cure.
9. Cementation-Crowns, etc. Mix equal parts of the shade base and catalyst until the mix is uniform, approximately 30 seconds.
10. Prepare to pass the cement and the PFI to the dentist for placement.
11. Remove the excess once the cement has gelled.
12. For veneers, place the Lute-It Cement base (light-cured) on the restoration, then place the veneer, and then light-cure for 10 seconds. Remove the excess and then light-cure for 40 seconds.

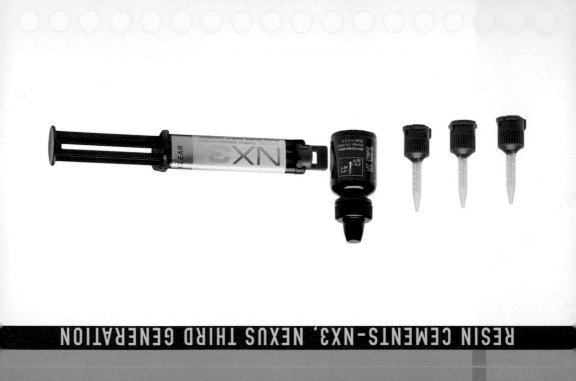

MANUFACTURER:
Kerr-Sybron

USE:
- Cement for veneers
- Adhesive for ceramic, porcelain, metal, and resin crowns, inlays/onlays, and bridges
- Excellent adhesion to cad/cam block
- Can be used for core buildup

COMPOSITION:
- Uncured methacrylate ester monomers
- Nonhazardous inert mineral fillers, stabilizers, activators, and radiopaque agent

PROPERTIES:
- Simple delivery dual mix
- Unmatched esthetics, high translucency, and excellent color stability

- Versatility in light-cure and dual-cure
- Try in gels with both techniques
- Desirable non-slumping, easy control and cleanup
- Contains fluoride
- Highly radiopaque
- Nano-filled for easy placement and polishing
- Excellent bond strength

OSHA INFORMATION:

- May cause irritation to the eyes and skin
- May cause respiratory irritation
- Do not ingest

MIXING AND SETTING TIME:

- Automix system
- Work time is 2 to 3 minutes.
- Cleanup time is 2 to 3 minutes.
- Finishing and polishing time for self-cure approximately 4 to 5 minutes.

DIRECTIONS:

1. The dentist will choose a shade by using the try-in gels to see the optimum match.

2. The try-in gel is then rinsed off thoroughly and the tooth is lightly air-dried.

3. The restoration is prepared by sandblasting or micro-etching, then rinsed thoroughly, and dried.

4. Place the Silane to the internal surface of composite, ceramic, or porcelain restorations and air-dry gently. If the restoration is metal, a bonding agent is used.

5. The tooth is cleaned and prepared with Optibond All-in-One bonding agent. The bonding agent is placed in a well and an applicator is used to place the material on the tooth. Scrub the first coat for 20 seconds. (Note various bonding agents could also be used.)

6. Apply a second coat and scrub for 20 seconds, dry the adhesive with air, and then light-cure for 10 seconds.

7. Attach a new mixing tip to the dual-cured syringe and dispense a small amount of cement on a paper pad. It is now ready to pass to the dentist.
8. The cement is dispensed on the tooth or in the restoration. The restoration is then seated on the tooth.
9. Allow the excess cement to flow away from the tooth and then remove.
10. Light-cure all surfaces for 20 seconds each.
11. Remove the disposable tip from the syringe and discard. Place the cap back on the syringe for storage. Finish and polish the restoration.

RESIN CEMENTS-VARIOLINK (VERY SIMILAR TO PANAVIA-KURARAY AMERICA AND NEXUS 2 AND NEXUS 2 DUAL-SYRINGE-KERR)

MANUFACTURER:
Ivoclar Vivadent

USE:
- Adhesive luting for indirect restorations including crowns, bridges, inlays/onlays, and veneers made from translucent ceramics and composites and FRC
- Core buildups

COMPOSITION:
- BIS-GMA, inorganic fillers, fluoride, initiators, stabilizers and pigments, and benzoyl peroxide

PROPERTIES:

- High degree of strength
- Highest radiopacity
- Light- and dual-cured
- Six shades and three degrees of translucency for very good optical properties
- Two consistencies
- High abrasion resistance

OSHA PRECAUTIONS:

- Irritating to the eyes and skin
- Irritating to the respiratory system

MIXING AND SETTING TIME:

- Mixing time is 10 seconds.
- Working time is 3 1/2 minutes.
- Material is light-cured to set.

DIRECTIONS:

1. The Variolink II base may be used alone and light-cured to set with some restoration such as veneers. Ceramic and composite restorations require the use of both the base and the catalyst for the self-curing and light-curing around the margins.
2. Prepare the restoration according to manufacturer's instructions.
3. After the temporary has been removed and the dentist has tried in restoration, the tooth is rinsed and dried.
4. An etchant is applied and then the tooth is rinsed thoroughly and gently dried. A bonding agent is placed according to manufacturer's instructions.
5. Dispense equal portions of the base and catalyst material on a paper pad and mix for 10 seconds until the mix is uniform and smooth.
6. The mix is applied to the tooth with a brush or a spatula. The restoration is seated and the excess cement should be removed after tacking the margins by light-curing them for 10 to 20 seconds.
7. Light-cure all segments of the sealed restoration for 40 seconds each.

TEMPORARY ZINC OXIDE-EUGENOL CEMENTS—
TEMPBOND, TEMPBOND NE, AND TEMPBOND CLEAR

MANUFACTURER:
Kerr

USE:
- To cement temporary restorations
- Temporary cement for trial cementations

COMPOSITION:
- TempBond-Accelerator is eugenol and oil of cloves.
- Base is zinc oxide, mineral oil, and cornstarch.
- TempBond NE-Accelerator is resin, ortho ethocybenzoic acid, carnauba wax, and octanic acid.
- Base is zinc oxide, mineral oil, and cornstarch.
- TempBond Clear-Resin-based, uncured urethane diacrylate ester monomer, mineral fillers, activators, and fillers

PROPERTIES:
- TempBond—Flows easily
- Strong enough for temporary cementation

- Withstands mastication forces
- Seals the margins and prevents leakage
- Easy to mix and clean up
- Easy to remove
- Matches dentin color
- TempBond NE will not interfere with the polymerization of resin cements and acrylic temporaries. It has the same flow and retentive qualities.
- There are three delivery systems: two-paste, automix syringe, and unidose packets.
- Unidose packets are ideal to give patients who are traveling in case they lose their temporary.
- TempBond Clear has the same properties as the TempBond and is also a dual-cure material.

OSHA PRECAUTIONS:

- May be irritating to the eyes and skin
- Irritating to the respiratory system, remove the patient to fresh air
- If ingested, contact a physician

MIXING AND SETTING TIME:
- Mixing time is 30 seconds.
- Working time is 1 1/2 minutes.
- Setting time is 7 minutes for TempBond and TempBond NE, and 5 1/2 minutes for TempBond Clear.
- Note: To accelerate the set with the TempBond Clear, light-cure all surfaces for 20 seconds.

DIRECTIONS:
Tube or Paste

1. Dispense equal lengths of the base and accelerator on the mixing pad that is provided. Length and size is determined by the size of the temporary restoration.
2. Replace the caps tightly.
3. Mix for approximately 30 seconds until the mix is smooth, creamy, and uniform in color.
4. Wipe off the spatula and using a PFI, place TempBond cement on the tooth or temporary restoration.

5. Firmly seat the restoration in the mouth and once the material is set, remove the excess cement with a scaler.

Unidose

1. Using scissors, cut along the dotted line.
2. Squeeze the material on a mixing pad.
3. Mix for 30 seconds.
4. Continue as described with the tube techniques.

Syringe

1. Remove the cap from the syringe and dispense a small amount on a gauze or paper pad.
2. Place the automix tip on the syringe and turn until locked in place.
3. Material is ready to dispense directly into the temporary or on the tooth.

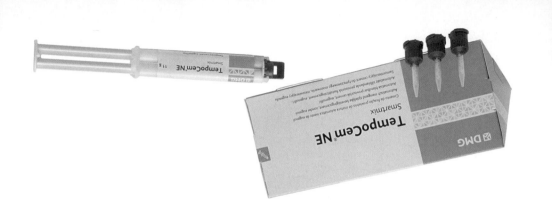

TEMPORARY ZINC OXIDE-EUGENOL
CEMENTS-TEMPOCEM, TEMPOCEM NE,
TEMPOCEM NE SMARTMIX

MANUFACTURER:
Zenith/DMG

USE:
- Temporary cement for attaching all kinds of temporaries, such as crowns, bridges, inlays, and onlays

COMPOSITION:
- TempoCem—Catalyst consists of natural resins, eugenol, and additives.
- TempoCem NE formulas—Catalyst consists of natural resins, fatty acids, and additives.
- Base for both materials is zinc oxide, paraffin, and additives. The non-eugenol materials are used with resin and resin-reinforced glass ionomer materials.

PROPERTIES:
- Comes in eugenol and non-eugenol formulas
- Resists forces of mastication

- Securely retains the temporary restoration
- Easy to remove
- Resistant to saliva and protects the gingival tissues
- Radiopaque on X-rays
- Easy flow and no heat generated
- Protects against thermal sensitivity
- Comes in a variety of forms with automixing and direct dispensing

OSHA PRECAUTIONS:

- May be irritating to the eyes and skin
- Irritating to the respiratory system, remove patient to fresh air
- If ingested, contact a physician

MIXING AND SETTING TIME:

- No mixing is required.
- Working time is 1 minute.
- Setting time is from 1 to 3 minutes.

DIRECTIONS:

Smartmix

1. Prepare the tooth and the temporary by rinsing thoroughly and air-drying.
2. Remove the cap from the Smartmix syringe and dispense a test amount on a paper pad or gauze.
3. Place a disposable syringe tip on the syringe and twist to secure.
4. Dispense the amount needed on the tooth or in the temporary restoration.
5. Place the temporary on the tooth and apply pressure until the material has set.
6. Remove any excess material from the margins.

Cartridge

1. Prepare the tooth and temporary by rinsing thoroughly and air-drying.
2. Prepare the DMG Type 25 Applicator Gun by releasing the small lever in the back and make sure the slide is in position.

3. Lift the top level and slide the cartridge into place. The notch on the bottom of the cartridge aligns with the notch in the gun. Push down firmly to lock into place.

4. Remove the cap on the cartridge and dispense a small portion. Place the disposable cannula on the cartridge by lining up the notches. Twist it clockwise 90 degrees to lock into place.

5. Pull the trigger to dispense the material.

6. When finished, remove the cannula and replace the storage cap on the end of the capsule.

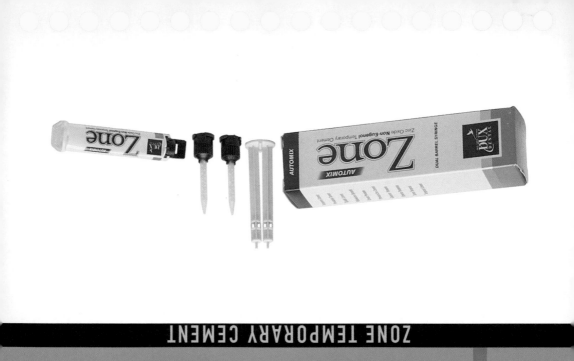

MANUFACTURER:
Dux Cadco Dental Products

USE:
- Temporary cement for all provisionals
- Temporary cement for trial cementation of permanent restorations for evaluation purposes

COMPOSITION:
- Crystalline zinc oxide preparation

PROPERTIES:
- Smooth
- Rigid setting
- Consistent retention
- Easy removal and clean up
- Compatible with provisional materials
- Does not soften, craze, or discolor polycarbonate or acrylic crown forms
- Kind to the tooth

- Available in tubes, unidose, and syringe
- Non-eugenol

OSHA PRECAUTIONS:

- May be irritating to the eyes and skin
- Irritating to the respiratory system, remove patient to fresh air
- If ingested, contact a physician

MIXING AND SETTING TIME:

- Mixing time is 30 seconds.
- Working time is approximately 1 1/2 minutes.
- Setting time is 5 to 7 minutes.

DIRECTIONS:

Standard Two Tubes

1. Dispense equal lengths of the base and accelerator on the mixing pad that is provided. Length and size is determined by the size of the temporary restoration.

2. Replace the caps tightly.

3. Mix for approximately 30 seconds until the mix is smooth, creamy, and uniform in color.
4. Wipe off spatula and using a PFI, place Zone cement on the tooth or temporary restoration.
5. Firmly seat the restoration in the mouth and once the material is set, remove the excess cement with a scaler.

Unidose
1. Using scissors, cut along the dotted line.
2. Squeeze the material on a mixing pad.
3. Mix for 30 seconds.
4. Place in temporary restoration with a PFI. Seat the restoration in the mouth and hold in place until set. Remove excess cement.

Automix Syringe and Auto-Aspirating Dual-Cartridge, Single-Plunger Syringe
1. Remove the cap from the syringe and dispense a small amount on a gauze or paper pad to be sure the materials are mixing evenly.
2. Place the automix tip on the syringe and turn until locked in place.
3. Material is ready to dispense directly into the temporary or on the tooth.

TEMPORARY RESTORATIVE MATERIALS-IRM
(INTERMEDIATE RESTORATIVE MATERIAL)
AND IRM CAPS

MANUFACTURER:
Dentsply Caulk

USE:
- Restoration of primary teeth if permanent teeth are within two years of eruption
- Restorative emergencies
- Caries management for Class I and II restorations lasting up to one year
- Public health care programs and dental school clinic application

COMPOSITION:
- Powder—polymer-reinforced zinc oxide
- Liquid—eugenol material and acetic acid
- Comes in a powder/liquid and capsules

PROPERTIES:
- Fairly strong
- Low abrasion qualities

- Low solubility
- Prevents microleakage
- Fairly easy to mix and clean up
- Easy to place
- Material can be carved with a small round bur when hardened, if necessary.

OSHA PRECAUTIONS:

- May be irritating to the eyes and skin
- Irritating to the respiratory system, remove the patient to fresh air
- If ingested, contact a physician

MIXING AND SETTING TIME:

- Mixing time for the powder/liquid is 1 minute.
- Mixing time for the capsule is 8 to 30 seconds depending on the amalgamator. Mix at high speed.
- Setting time is 5 minutes from start to finish.

DIRECTIONS:

IRM Powder/Liquid

1. Prepare the tooth by rinsing and drying completely. Place a liner if needed.
2. Powder/Liquid-Fluff the powder and using the scoop provided, measure 1 level scoop with the spatula and place on the paper pad.
3. Dispense 1 drop of liquid and replace the cap immediately to prevent evaporation. (When the liquid reaches the discard level marked on the bottle, it should be discarded.)
4. Bring 1/2 of the powder into the liquid and mix quickly and thoroughly.
5. Bring remaining powder into the mix in 2 or 3 increments and spatulate thoroughly.
6. Once all the powder is in the mix, continue mixing for 5 to 10 seconds. Mix will become smooth and adaptable. Completely mix in 1 minute.
7. IRM is now ready to place.

IRM-Caps

1. To activate the IRM capsule, hold it vertical. Hold the bottom half and turn the top firmly until you feel a snap as the liquid is released.
2. Continue to tighten to be sure it is seated.
3. Place the capsule in an amalgamator and mix for a designated amount of time.
4. Once mixed, remove the bottom lid (called the press cap) and remove the mixed IRM.
5. It may be placed on a paper pad for dispensing or directly into the tooth.

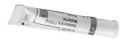

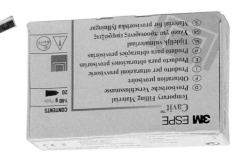

TEMPORARY RESTORATIVE MATERIALS-CAVIT AND
CAVIT G

MANUFACTURER:
3M ESPE

USE:
- Temporary filling material for Class I and II

COMPOSITION:
- Zinc oxide
- Calcium sulfate
- Barium sulfate and talc
- Ethylene BIS diacetate and zinc sulfate
- Poly(vinyl acetate)

PROPERTIES:
- High surface hardness
- Simple to apply
- Slight expansion seals margins
- Light-cured
- Comes in a tube or jar

OSHA PRECAUTIONS:

- May be irritating to the eyes and skin
- Irritating to the respiratory system, remove patient to fresh air
- If ingested, contact a physician

MIXING AND SETTING TIME:

- No mixing
- The hardening process begins within a few minutes and the patient should be advised to avoid chewing pressure for about 2 hours after application.

DIRECTIONS:

1. Remove the cap and use the sharp end to puncture the metal end of the tube on the first time used.
2. Squeeze from the bottom of the tube to extrude a small amount of material. Replace the cap immediately. Use a PFI to take the Cavit from the tube and place in the cavity. If additional material is required, use a clean instrument to remove what is needed.

3. Wipe the excess from the instrument with gauze and continue filling the cavity. The cavity should be moist. Once the material is placed, have the patient bite down and then remove the excess material.
4. The hardening process begins a few minutes after placement.
5. Patient should avoid chewing pressure for about 2 hours after application.
6. Cavit G is applied following the same steps.

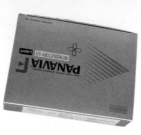
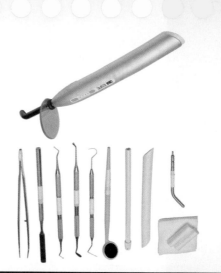
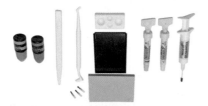

PROCEDURE: PERMANENT CEMENTATION OF A PFM CROWN WITH PANAVIA F 2.0 DUAL-CURE DENTAL RESIN ADHESIVE

This procedure is performed by the dentist and the dental assistant at chairside.

EQUIPMENT AND SUPPLIES:

- Basic setup
- Air/water syringe tip, HVE, and salvia ejector
- Cotton rolls and 2×2 gauze sponges
- Spoon excavator
- Cement spatula
- Plastic filling instrument (PFI)
- Sandblaster or microetcher
- Panavia F 2.0 Dental Adhesive System
- Curing light
- PPE worn by the dental assistant

DIRECTIONS:

After the patient is seated, the temporary is removed and the crown is tried on for any adjustments before cementation. The crown and tooth are then prepared as follows before cementation:

1. The internal surface of the crown is sandblasted or micro-etched, then rinsed and dried.

2. Dispense 1 to 2 drops of alloy primer into the mixing well and prepare a clean applicator for placement. Place the primer on the inside of the clean crown.

3. The dental assistant then dispenses equal amounts of the ED Primer II A & B (the ED Primer II initiates the set of the cement) into a mixing well, prepares a clean applicator, and mixes the material together. The dental assistant passes the applicator to the dentist and the primer is placed on the tooth. Wait for 30 seconds and then the assistant gently air-dries the tooth.

4. The assistant dispenses equal amounts of the paste A & B on a paper pad and mixes the material for 20 seconds and then passes the PFI to the dentist and holds the paper pad for the dentist to place the paste mixture into the crown.

5. The crown is firmly seated on the tooth and the excess cement is removed. In some cases the excess margins are light-cured for 2 to 3 seconds for easy cleanup.

6. After the excess cement is removed the margins are light-cured for 5 to 20 seconds depending on the curing light or Oxyguard II is applied to the margins for self-curing in 3 minutes.
7. The dental assistant rinses and dries the area around the crown and dismisses the patient.

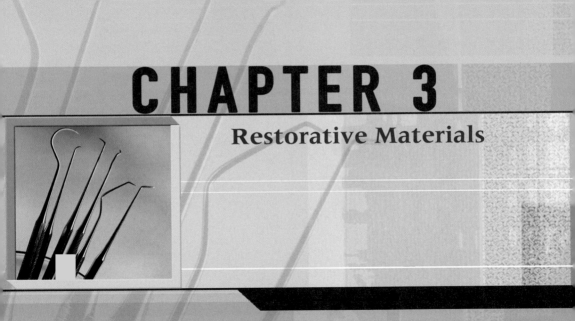

CHAPTER 3

Restorative Materials

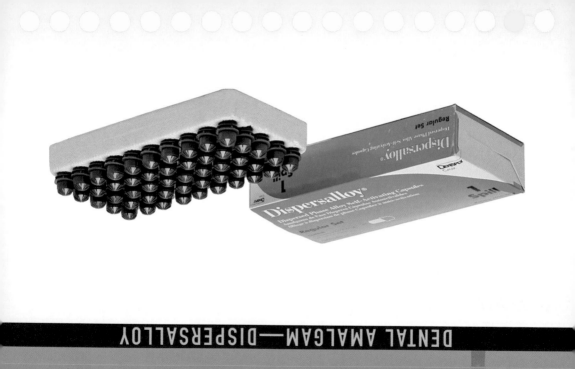
DENTAL AMALGAM—DISPERSALLOY

MANUFACTURER:
Dentsply Caulk

USE:
- Stress-bearing restorative material for posterior teeth (Class I and II)

COMPOSITION:
- Alloy powder contains silver, tin, copper, and zinc (Contains lathe-cut particles and silver/copper eutectic spheres that bond tin to copper)
- Mercury

PROPERTIES:
- Strong and durable material
- Corrosion resistant
- Reduced ditching
- Self-activating capsules
- Lustrous finish

- Strong margin integrity
- Comes in single, double, and triple spills
- Comes in regular and fast set

OSHA PRECAUTIONS:

- Material can cause irritation to the skin and eyes.
- Material may be irritating to respiratory system if powder is inhaled.
- If ingested, it may cause irritation, vomiting, and diarrhea.

MIXING AND SETTING TIME:

- Mixing time depends on type of amalgamator, regular set or fast set, and number of spills. Refer to manufacturer's instructions (usually between 6 and 14 seconds).
- Setting time is 4 to 5 minutes for initial set and 24 hours before polishing.

DIRECTIONS:

1. The tooth is prepared and the necessary liners, bonding agents, and matrix are placed.
2. The amalgam capsule is self-activating so it is simply placed in the amalgamator.
3. The mixing and trituration speed is set according to manufacturer's instructions.
4. Follow the guidelines to achieve the proper amalgam mix consistency.
5. The amalgam mix is removed from the capsule and placed into an amalgam well, dappen dish, or squeeze cloth for loading into an amalgam carrier.
6. Load both ends of the carrier and pass to the dentist for placement and condensation.
7. Repeat loading the carrier as the dentist requires.
8. Place the amalgam scraps in well-sealed container. Regulations for disposal must be followed.

- Comes in five settings: slow, regular, fast, extra-carving time (ECT), and slow carving (SC)
- Comes in 1, 2, 3, and 5 spills

OSHA PRECAUTIONS:
- Material can cause irritation to the skin and eyes.
- Material may be irritating to respiratory system if powder is inhaled.
- If ingested, it may cause irritation, vomiting, and diarrhea.

MIXING AND SETTING TIME:
- Mixing time depends on type of amalgamator.
- Setting time is 2 1/2 to 6 minutes depending on type of mix.
- Carving time is 5 1/2 to 9 minutes depending on type of mix.

DIRECTIONS:
1. The tooth is prepared and the necessary liners, bonding agents and matrix are placed.

2. The amalgam capsule is self-activating so it is simply placed in the amalgamator.
3. The mixing and trituration speed is set according to the manufacturer's instructions.
4. Follow the guidelines to achieve the proper amalgam mix consistency.
5. The amalgam mix is removed from the capsule and placed into an amalgam well, dappen dish, or squeeze cloth for loading into an amalgam carrier.
6. Load both ends of the carrier and pass to the dentist for placement and condensation.
7. Repeat loading the carrier as the dentist requires.
8. Place the amalgam scraps in a well-sealed container. Regulations for disposal must be followed.

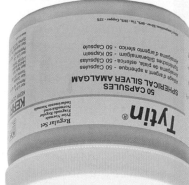

Tytin®

50 CAPSULES
SPHERICAL SILVER AMALGAM

Alliage d'argent à sphérique - 50 Capsules
Amalgama de plata, esférica - 50 Cápsulas
Sphärisches Silberamalgam - 50 Kapseln
Amalgama d'argento sferico - 50 Capsule

Alloy Composition: Silver - 60%, Tin - 28%, Copper - 12%

KERR

Regular Set
Prise Normale Regular
Fraguado Regular
Normalhärtend
Indurimento Normale

MANUFACTURER:
Kerr

USE:
- Posterior restorative material

COMPOSITION:
- Ternary alloy with high copper content
- Spherical particles of silver, tin, and copper
- Lower mercury content

PROPERTIES:
- Excellent clinical performance
- Higher in strength and lower in creep than other amalgams
- Very smooth surface
- Easy to place, carve and accepts immediate polishing 8 minutes in Class I restorations
- Comes in slow and regular set and single, double, and triple spill

- Each capsule is ensured to have the perfect ratio with pouched mercury.
- Reliable and consistent mixes
- Works with any amalgamator
- Self-activating
- Is color-coded

OSHA PRECAUTIONS:

- Material can cause irritation to the skin and eyes.
- Material may be irritating to respiratory system if powder is inhaled.
- If ingested, it may cause irritation, vomiting, and diarrhea.

MIXING AND SETTING TIME:

- Mixing time—follow the manufacturer's instructions (7 to 8 1/2 seconds)
- Setting time is 4 to 5 minutes for the initial set.

DIRECTIONS:

1. The tooth is prepared and the necessary liners, bonding agents, and matrix are placed.
2. The amalgam capsule is self-activating so it is simply placed in the amalgamator.
3. The mixing and trituration speed is set according to manufacturer's instructions.
4. Follow the guidelines to achieve the proper amalgam mix consistency.
5. The amalgam mix is removed from the capsule and placed into an amalgam well, dappen dish, or squeeze cloth for loading into an amalgam carrier.
6. Load both ends of the carrier and pass to the dentist for placement and condensation.
7. Repeat loading the carrier as the dentist requires.
8. Place the amalgam scraps in a well-sealed container. Regulations for disposal must be followed.

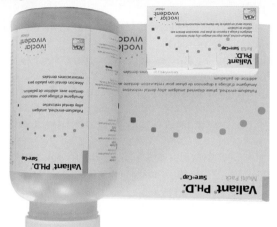

DENTAL AMALGAM—VALIANT AMALGAM, VALIANT PH.D., VALIANT SNAP-SET

MANUFACTURER:
Ivoclar Vivadent

USE:
- Posterior restorative material Class I and II

COMPOSITION:
- Valiant and Valiant Snap-Set—Spherical amalgam alloy with high copper content and palladium added plus mercury
- Valiant Ph.D Amalgam—Phase-dispersed amalgam with palladium enriched and with lower mercury content

PROPERTIES:
- Higher early strengths
- Corrosion resistance
- Smooth carving and burnishing
- Specially designed capsules that are ultrasonically welded for increased safety and efficiency
- Valiant Snap-Set has a faster setting time.

- Valiant Ph.D has a finer particle size for smoother carving, faster wetting, faster setting, and denser amalgam mass.
- All come in single, double, and triple spills.

OSHA PRECAUTIONS:

- Material can cause irritation to the skin and eyes.
- Material may be irritating to the respiratory system if powder is inhaled.
- If ingested, call a physician immediately.

MIXING AND SETTING TIME:

- Mixing time—follow the manufacturer's instructions (7 to 8 1/2 seconds).
- Setting time is 4 to 5 minutes for initial set.

DIRECTIONS:

1. The tooth is prepared and the necessary liners, bonding agents, and matrix are placed.

2. The amalgam capsule is self-activating so it is simply placed in the amalgamator.
3. The mixing and trituration speed is set according to manufacturer's instructions.
4. Follow the guidelines to achieve the proper amalgam mix consistency.
5. The amalgam mix is removed from the capsule and placed into an amalgam well, dappen dish, or squeeze cloth for loading into an amalgam carrier.
6. Load both ends of the carrier and pass to the dentist for placement and condensation.
7. Repeat loading the carrier as the dentist requires.
8. Place the amalgam scraps in a well-sealed container. Regulations for disposal must be followed.

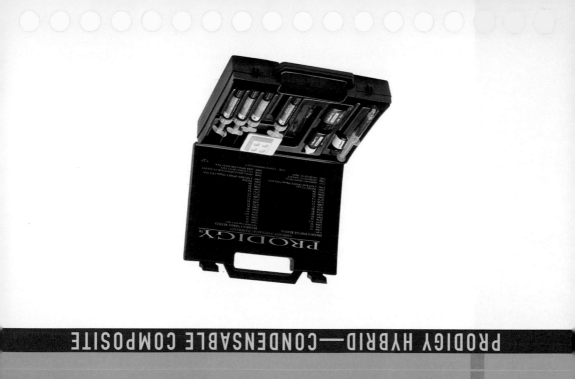

PRODIGY HYBRID—CONDENSABLE COMPOSITE

MANUFACTURER:
Kerr

USE:
- Primarily used for Class I and Class II posterior restorations
- Can be used for all classes of restorations

COMPOSITION:
- Hybrid composite resin with uncured methacrylate ester monomers
- Mineral fillers, activators, and fillers

PROPERTIES:
- Packable application
- Low shrinkage
- High esthetic quality
- Margin integrity
- Easy to use with proven system

- Can be bulk cured
- Proven filler technology

OSHA PRECAUTIONS:
- May be irritating to the skin with repeated and prolonged exposure
- Irritating to the eyes
- May be irritating if inhaled repeatedly
- Should not be ingested

MIXING AND SETTING TIME:
- No mixing is required. The material comes in unidose tips.
- Material is light–cured.

DIRECTIONS:
1. Select the shade of the tooth under natural light.
2. Tooth is prepared by the dentist.
3. Place OptiBond Solo Plus following manufacturer's instructions.
4. Light-cure the bonding agent.

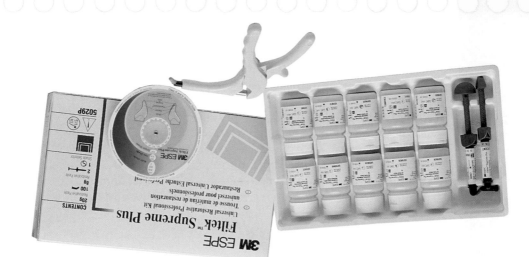

5. Place OptiGuard Surface Sealant according to manufacturer's instructions.
6. Place a new tip on the etchant syringe and place the etchant.
7. Leave the etchant in place for 10 to 15 seconds, then rinse and air–dry.
8. Place the matrix.
9. Select the shade of material and place the unidose tip in the unidose gun.
10. Apply the material directly into the cavity and condense; repeat this procedure and light-cure each layer for 20 seconds.
11. After polymerization, remove the excess material and finish with diamond burs, stones, and discs.

MANUFACTURER:
3M-ESPE

USE:
- Designed for anterior and posterior restorations
- Core buildups
- Splinting
- Indirect restorations including inlays, onlays, and veneers

COMPOSITION:
- Nanocomposite
- Bis-GMA, UDMA, TEGDMA, and Bis-EMA resins
- Between 72.5% and 78.5% filler

PROPERTIES:
- Highly regarded physical properties
- Excellent clinical properties
- Visible-light-activated material
- Comes in a variety of shades that blend easily

- Non-slumping and non-sticky
- Strong and dependable
- Wear comparable to enamel
- Also available as a flowable Filtek Supreme Plus Flowable
- Most shades are radiopaque

OSHA PRECAUTIONS:

- May cause eye irritation
- May cause skin irritation
- May cause problems if ingested

MIXING AND SETTING TIME:

- No mixing is required.
- Material is light–cured to set.

DIRECTIONS:

1. Before the tooth is prepared, select the shade under natural light.
2. The tooth is then prepared by the dentist.
3. A liner may be placed and then the matrix is positioned.

4. Follow manufacturer's instructions regarding etching, priming and adhesive application, and curing.
5. Dispense the composite as follows: Syringe—dispense necessary amount of material from the syringe onto a pad. If the material is not used immediately, protect it from light until used. Material is placed with PFI in incremental layers. Single-dose capsules—Place capsule into 3M-ESPE Restorative Dispenser, remove the cap, and pass to the dentist for placement.
6. Composite is placed in layers and light-cured after each layer.

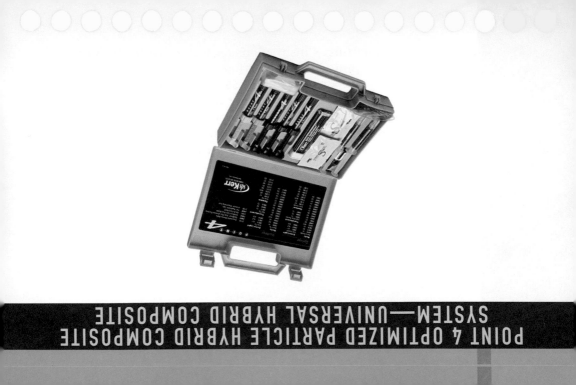

POINT 4 OPTIMIZED PARTICLE HYBRID COMPOSITE
SYSTEM—UNIVERSAL HYBRID COMPOSITE

MANUFACTURER:
Kerr

USE:
- Suitable for all classes of cavity preparations

COMPOSITION:
- Composite resin with 77% inorganic filler

PROPERTIES:
- Sixteen body shades, eight opaque shades, and three translucent shades
- All shades are radiopaque.
- Polishes to a smooth, lustrous finish
- Hybrid strength
- Bridges the gap between the microfill and hybrid composites
- Quick and easy to use
- True chameleon effect and blends with adjacent teeth

OSHA PRECAUTIONS:

- May be irritating to the skin with repeated and prolonged exposure
- Irritating to the eyes
- May be irritating if inhaled repeatedly
- Should not be ingested

MIXING AND SETTING TIMES:

- No mixing is required.
- Material is light-cured to set.

DIRECTIONS:

1. Prepare the etchant syringe and place the etchant in the cavity preparation for 15 seconds.
2. Rinse and dry lightly.
3. Apply OptiBond Solo Plus on enamel and dentin for 15 seconds using a light brushing motion. Lightly air-dry for 3 seconds and light-cure for 20 seconds.

4. Place the unidose base tip in the dispensing gun and pass to the dentist. Light-cure each layer for 20 seconds.
5. Place the unidose translucency tip in the dispensing gun and pass to the dentist. Light-cure after placement for 20 seconds.

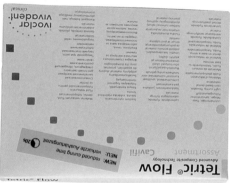

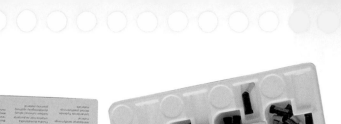

MANUFACTURER:
Ivoclar Vivadent

USE:
- Class V restorations (cervical caries, root erosion, wedge-shaped defects)
- Anterior restorations (Class III and IV)
- Small posterior restorations
- Extended fissure sealing in molars and premolars
- Blocking out of undercuts
- Adhesive cementation of ceramic and composite restorations

COMPOSITION:
- Monomer matrix of Bis-GMA, urethane, dimethacrylate, and triethylene glycol dimethacrylate, and 68% inorganic filler particles

PROPERTIES:

- Low viscosity permits optimum wetting of the tooth.
- A variety of shades are available for outstanding esthetics.
- Has fluoride release
- Radiopaque
- Easy to use and variety of applications

OSHA PRECAUTIONS:

- May be irritating to the skin
- Irritating to the eyes

MIXING AND SETTING TIMES:

- Material comes in single-use cartridges and syringe form.
- Material is light-cured to set.

DIRECTIONS:

1. The tooth has been prepared and the pulp protection and bonding agent are placed according to manufacturer's instructions.

2. Tetric Flow Cavifil cartridges are placed in the dispensing gun or Luer-lock applicator tips are placed on the Tetric Flow syringe.
3. The material is applied directly into the cavity preparation.
4. Light-cure each increment for 20 seconds.

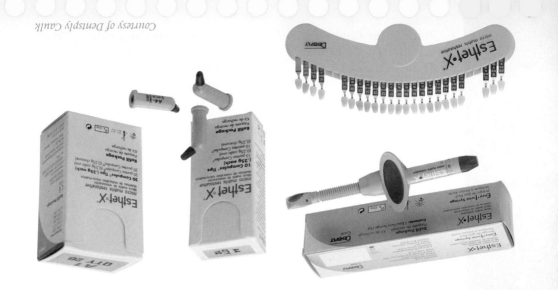

ESTHET X—MICRO MATRIX RESTORATIVE MATERIAL

MANUFACTURER:
Dentsply Caulk

USE:
- Esthetic restorative material for all cavity classes
- For primary and permanent dentition

COMPOSITION:
- Dimethacrylate resin (urethane modified Bis-GMA)
- Inorganic fillers (including silica, barium boron fluoro alumino silicate glass)
- Colorants

PROPERTIES:
- Outstanding physical properties
- Long working time
- High fracture toughness for strength and durability
- Radiopaque
- High wear resistance

- Adapts well to margins
- No patient sensitivity
- Low shrinkage
- Brilliant polish
- Optimum handling
- Comes with detailed shade guide
- Optimized 31 shades and 3 opacities

OSHA PRECAUTIONS:
- Can be irritating to eyes and skin
- No inhalation irritation
- Probably not harmful if ingested

MIXING AND SETTING TIMES:
- No mixing is required. Materials come in single dose compules or easy-twist syringe.
- Materials are light-cured to set.

DIRECTIONS:

1. Easy-twist syringe—remove cap in a "snap-off" twist with lateral force.
2. Dispense the necessary amount of Esthet X material from the syringe on the paper pad by turning the handle clockwise. When finished dispensing the material, turn the handle counterclockwise and replace the cap.
3. Pre-dosed Esthet X compules—load by inserting the compule tips into the notched opening of the compule dispensing gun. Be sure the collar on the compules is inserted first.
4. Remove the tip cover; the material is now ready to be dispensed.
5. Light-cure each area of the restoration for 20 seconds. The restoration may be placed in increments and will need to be light-cured after each layer.

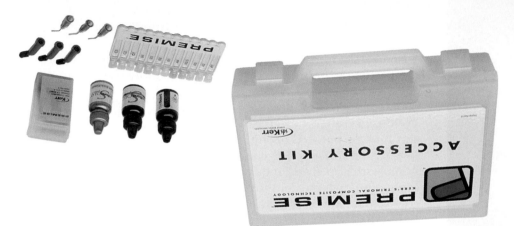

PREMISE UNIVERSAL NANO-RESTORATIVE
MATERIAL AND PREMISE FLOWABLE

MANUFACTURER:
Kerr

USE:
- Universal for all restoration on the anterior and posterior teeth
- Flowable is also used as pit and fissure sealants, repair of enamel defects, repair of porcelain restorations, minor occlusal buildups in nonstress areas, and incisal abrasions.

COMPOSITION:
- Resin: ethoxylated Bis-GMA, triethylene glycol dimethacrylate, light-cured initators and stabilizers
- Three fillers: prepolymerizable filler, barium glass, silica nanoparticles (84% filler)
- Polymerizable organophosphate dispersant

PROPERTIES:

- Universal material—ultra-low shrinkage
- Universal application with strength for the posterior teeth and esthetics for anterior teeth
- Three different fillers to improve this nano-restorative material
- Unmatched handling
- Comes in a variety of shades including body shades, translucent shades, and packable shades
- High polish and gloss characteristics
- Flowable material flows easily but holds its shape, excellent mechanical strength, low shrinkage, high polishability and wearability

OSHA PRECAUTIONS:

- Prolonged or repeated exposure may cause irritation to the skin.
- May cause irritation to the eyes

- Prolonged or excessive inhalation may cause irritation to the respiratory tract.
- May be harmful if swallowed

MIXING AND SETTING TIME:
- There is no mixing time. The universal comes in unidose tips and the flowable comes in a syringe.
- Both materials are light-cured to set.

DIRECTIONS:
Universal Premise
1. Apply self-etching bonding system following manufacturer's instructions.
2. Place the unidose tip of the selected shade into the dispensing gun.
3. Pass to the dentist and prepare the curing light.

4. Light-cure for 5 to 20 seconds depending on the curing light after each increment is placed.

5. When finished, remove the unidose tip from the gun and dispose.

Flowable Premise

1. Apply self-etching bonding system following manufacturer's instructions.

2. Place disposable tip on selected shade of Premise Flowable and secure.

3. Pass to the dentist and prepare the curing light.

4. The dentist will flow the material into the cavity preparation and place in layers. Light-cure for 5 to 20 seconds depending on the curing light.

5. Restoration is finished and polished.

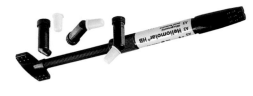

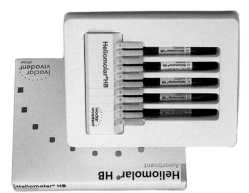

HELIOMOLAR HB—PACKABLE MICROFILLED RESTORATIVE MATERIAL

MANUFACTURER:
Ivoclar Vivadent

USE:
- Microfill composite for the posterior region
- Restorations in primary teeth

COMPOSITION:
- Monomer matrix of Bis-GMA, urethane dimethacrylate, decandiol dimeth acrylate
- Fillers include copolymer, silicone dioxide, yetterbium trifluoride
- Total amount of inorganic fillers is approximately 66%.
- Catalysts, stabilizers, and pigments

PROPERTIES:
- Highly viscous packable material
- Nine shades to choose from
- Highly radiopaque

- Low wear value
- Polishes to a long-lasting high gloss

OSHA PRECAUTIONS:

- May be irritating to the eyes and the skin
- No problems anticipated if small amount of material is ingested
- If irritating when inhaled, move to fresh air.

MIXING AND SETTING TIME:

- There is no mixing. Material comes in a syringe or a Cavifill.
- Material is light-cured for 20 seconds for each increment.

DIRECTIONS:

1. The tooth is conditioned and bonding agent is applied following manufacturer's instructions.
2. Prepare and coat the cavity with a layer of Heliomolar flow.
3. Heliomolar comes in either a syringe or a Cavifill. Prepare the syringe by removing the cap and dispensing the selected shade on a pad.

4. Hold the pad and pass the plugger/condensing composite instrument.
5. Cavifills—place the selected shade of Cavifill and place it into the dispensing gun.
6. Secure the Cavifill and remove the tip. Pass to the dentist for placement.
7. Heliomolar is placed in increments and each increment is light-cured after placement for 20 seconds.
8. Several shades may be used to achieve the desired results.

TETRIC—MICROHYBRID COMPOSITE RESTORATIVE MATERIAL

MANUFACTURER:
Ivoclar Vivadent

USE:
- All classes of restoration anterior and posterior (Class I, II, III, IV, and V)
- Veneering of discolored anterior teeth
- Preventive restoration in premolars and molars
- Splinting of mobile teeth
- Repairing ceramic and composite veneers

COMPOSITION:
- Monomer matrix of Bis-GMA, urethane dimethacrylate, triethylene glycol dimethacrylate

- Fillers of barium glass, yetterbium trifluoride, highly dispersed silicon dioxide, spherical mixed dioxide (81% fill)
- Cataylists, stabilizers, and pigments

PROPERTIES:
- Good polishability
- Radiopacity is good.
- Continuous fluoride release
- High shade stability
- Easy handling
- Thirteen shades including one translucent and three opaque dentin shades

OSHA PRECAUTIONS:
- May be irritating to the eyes and the skin
- No problems anticipated if small amount of material is ingested
- If irritating when inhaled, move to fresh air.

MIXING AND SETTING TIME:

- There is no mixing. Material comes in a syringe or a Cavifill.
- Material is light-cured for 40 seconds for each increment.

DIRECTIONS:

1. Apply conditioner and bonding agent according to manufacturer's directions. Recommended to use product from the same manufacturer.
2. Tetric comes in either a syringe or a Cavifill. Prepare the syringe by removing the cap and dispensing the selected shade on a pad.
3. Hold the paper pad and pass the plugger/condensing composite instrument.
4. Cavifill—place the selected shade of Tetric and place it into the dispensing gun.
5. Secure the Cavifill in the dispensing gun and then remove the tip. Pass to the dentist for placement.

6. Tetric is placed in increments and each increment is light-cured after placement for 40 seconds.
7. Several shades may be used to achieve the desired results of matching the tooth coloring.

GLACIER—MICROFILLED HYBRID COMPOSITE

MANUFACTURER:
SDI

USE:
- Anterior and posterior esthetic restorations (Class I, II, III, IV, and V)
- Veneers
- Inlays/onlays
- Core buildups

COMPOSITION:
- Microfilled hybrid composite with strontium glass and amorphous silica
- Initiators, stabilizers, and pigments

PROPERTIES:
- High compressive strength
- Radiopaque
- Low shrinkage that reduces sensitivity and microleakage

- Wear resistant
- Non-stick and non-slump
- Polishes to a high luster

OSHA PRECAUTIONS:

- May be irritating to the eyes and the skin
- No problems anticipated if small amount of material is ingested
- If irritating when inhaled, move to fresh air.

MIXING AND SETTING TIMES:

- Material comes in a syringe or Complets. There is no mixing.
- Glacier is light-cured to set.

DIRECTIONS:

1. Etch the tooth for 20 seconds with 37% phosphoric etchant.
2. Rinse the tooth thoroughly and then remove excess moisture leaving the tooth moist.
3. Apply a bonding agent according to manufacturer's instruction and light-cure for 20 seconds.

4. Gently blow-dry for 2 seconds until glossy, then light-cure 20 seconds.
5. Prepare the syringe of the selected shade by removing the cap and placing a dispensing tip on the end. If using the Complets (compules), place the Complets in the Complets applicator and snap to secure. Remove the end from the Complets.
6. Pass to the dentist for placement. Light-cure after each increment is placed for 20 seconds.
7. Restoration is ready to finish and polish.

SIMILE NANO-HYBRID COMPOSITE

MANUFACTURER:
Pentron Clinical Technologies

USE:
- Esthetic restoration for both anterior and posterior teeth

COMPOSITION:
- A mixture of difunctional methacrylate of PCBis-GMA, Bis-GMA, UDMA, HDDMA, barium boron silicate glass, nano-particulated silica, zirconium silicate, photo initiator, accelerator, stabilizers, Silane, and pigments

PROPERTIES:
- Sculptable handling that will not stick to instruments
- Superior surface for easy polishability and retention of shine
- Low wear rates for long-lasting restoration
- Familiar shades that are easy to use

OSHA PRECAUTIONS:
- Irritating to the skin and eyes, rinse with plenty of water and contact medical attention
- If ingested, seek medical attention

MIXING AND SETTING TIME:
- No mixing is required.
- Light-cured to set.

DIRECTIONS:
1. Apply bonding agent according to manufacturer's instructions.
2. Select the syringe(s) of the desired shade and remove the tip.
3. Dispense material on paper pad and prepare for placement.

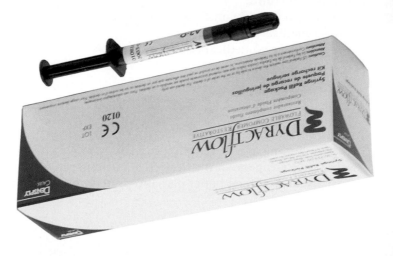

DYRACT EXTRA UNIVERSAL COMPOMER

MANUFACTURER:
Dentsply Caulk

USE:
- Direct esthetic restoration indicated for all cavity classifications (Class I through V)
- Anterior and posterior teeth

COMPOSITION:
- Polymerizable dimethacrylate resin—urethane dimethacrylate resin, trimethacrylate resin, carboxylic acid modified dimethacrylate, triethyleneglycol dimethacrylate, camphorquinone, ethyl–4 dimethylaminobenzoate, butylated hydroxy toluene
- UV stabilizer
- Strontium alumino sodium fluoro-silicate glass
- Colorants are inorganic iron oxides.

PROPERTIES:

- Improved physical properties—less sticky handling and increased working time
- Excellent wear resistant
- Fluoride release
- Shortened curing time
- Easier finishing and polishing to a high luster restoration
- Comes in a variety of shades
- Also comes in a flowable composition

OSHA PRECAUTIONS:

- May be irritating to the eyes
- May cause irritation to the skin
- Material is probably not harmful if swallowed

MIXING AND SETTING TIME:

- No mixing is required. Dyract comes in individual compule tips.
- Material is light-cured for 10 to 20 seconds.

DIRECTIONS:

1. Place 2 to 3 drops of self-etching adhesive into clean mixing well.
2. Apply generous amount with small applicator and scrub for 15 seconds, then repeat.
3. Spread the adhesive and then gently spread with air until there is no more flow of the material—about 5 seconds.
4. Light-cure at least 10 seconds and then immediately place the restoration.
5. The selected shade of Dyract Xtra compule tip is placed in the Compules Tips gun. Load by inserting the compules tips into the notched opening of the Compules Tips gun. Be sure the collar on the compules is inserted first.
6. The cap is removed and the material is ready for placement.
7. Dyract Xtra is placed in 2 mm increments and light-cured after each increment is placed for 10 to 20 seconds. This is repeated until restoration is completed.
8. Restoration is ready to finish and polish.

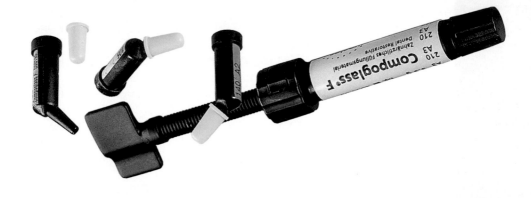

COMPOGLASS F—COMPOMER-BASED RESTORATIVE MATERIAL

MANUFACTURER:
Ivoclar Vivadent

USE:
- Restoration for deciduous teeth
- Class V (cervical caries, root erosion, and wedge-shaped defects)
- Class III restorations
- Intermediate Class I and II restorations

COMPOSITION:
- Monomer matrix of urethane dimethacrylate, tetraethylene glycol dimethacrylate, cycloatiphatic dicarboxylic acid dimethacrylate. Inorganic fillers—Ba-fluorosilicate glass, mixed oxides, yetterbium trifluoride (77% inorganic fillers). Catalysts, stabilizers, and pigments

PROPERTIES:
- Advantages of glass ionomer cements and light-cured composites
- Radiopaque

- Polishable
- Higher fluoride release
- High abrasion resistance
- Excellent bonding to enamel and dentin

OSHA PRECAUTIONS:

- Flush with water if material gets into the eyes
- May cause skin irritation—wash with water and soap
- No known problems if ingested
- Remove to fresh air if respiratory irritation

MIXING AND SETTING TIMES:

- No mixing is required.
- Light-cure to set

DIRECTIONS:

1. It is recommended to use a bonding agent from Ivoclar Vivadent.
2. Apply primer to the cavity preparation using a small applicator tip. Brush on for 30 seconds and then disperse excess liquid with strong stream of air until mobile liquid has disappeared.

3. Apply bonding agent with applicator tip. Using a gentle air stream, disperse evenly and light-cure for 10 seconds.
4. Load the Cavifil capsule into the dispensing gun and secure. Remove the cap.
5. Pass to the dentist for placement with a placement instrument such as the PFI. Material will be placed in increments and light-cured for 40 seconds after each increment is placed.
6. Close the Cavifil capsule after placement. Restoration is ready to finish.

GC FUJI IX GP-GLASS IONOMER RESTORATIVE MATERIAL

MANUFACTURER:
GC America

USE:
- Geriatric and pediatric restorations (Class I and II)
- Final restoration in non-stress areas
- Core-buildups
- Class V and root surface restorations
- Long-term temporaries

COMPOSITION:
- Glass Ionomer
- Liquid=polyacrylic acid
- Powder=polyacrylic acid and aluminosilicate glass

PROPERTIES:
- Easy to handle and packable
- Chemically bonds to tooth structure

- Cures extremely hard and is very wear resistant
- Fluoride release
- Non-sticky
- High compressive and flexural strength
- Placed and finished similar to amalgam

OSHA PRECAUTIONS:
- If ingested do not induce vomiting, give water and seek medical attention
- May be irritating to the eyes—flush with water for 15 minutes
- May be irritating to the skin—wash with soap and water

MIXING AND SETTING TIME:
- Two minute working time
- Self-cures in 2.5 minutes (4.5 minutes from start)

DIRECTIONS:
1. Rinse the cavity preparation and air dry gently.
2. Shade the capsule or tap on a hard surface to loosen the powder.

3. **Push the plunger in until it is even with the capsule or** immediately place capsule in the GC metal capsule activator and compress handle until it clicks. This activates the capsule.

4. Immediately place the activated capsule into an amalgamator and triturate for 10 seconds +/− the designated amount of time depending on the amalgamator/mixer.

5. Immediately remove the capsule from the amalgamator and place in the GC applier. Compress the handle for two clicks to be sure the material is ready. Remove the tip and pass to the dentist for placement.

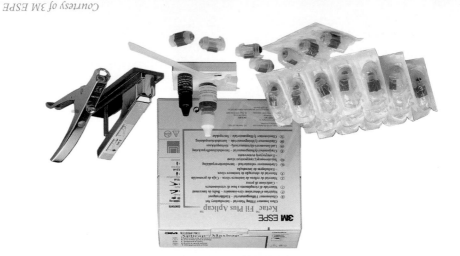

Courtesy of 3M ESPE

KETAC FIL PLUS APLICAP—GLASS IONOMER
RESTORATIVE MATERIAL

MANUFACTURER:
3M-ESPE

USE:
- Ideal for pediatric and geriatric patients
- Class III and V restorations
- Cervical defects
- Small Class I
- Core build-ups

COMPOSITION:
- Glass ionomer
- Powder=glass powder
- Liquid=water, polyethylene, polycarbonic acid and tartaric acid

PROPERTIES:
- High compressive strength
- Minimal abrasion
- Excellent surface hardness

- Fluoride release
- Bulk placement
- Chemical bonds to enamel and dentin
- Eight shades
- Tooth—like co-efficient of thermal expansion thus less shrinkage and microleakage
- Radiopaque

OSHA PRECAUTIONS:

- May be irritating to the skin and eyes
- Should not be ingested
- May cause upper respiratory irritation

MIXING AND SETTING TIME:

- Activating the Aplicap—2 seconds
- Mix the Aplicap for 8 to 10 seconds in a rotary mixer or an amalgamator
- Processing from start of mix is 1:30 minutes
- Setting from start of mix is 7 minutes

DIRECTIONS:

1. Prepare tooth according to manufacturer's instructions.
2. Rinse and gently dry the cavity preparation. Do not over dry.
3. Activate the Aplicap by placing it in the Aplicap Activator and squeezing the handle.
4. Remove Aplicap and immediately place in rotary mixer or amalgamator for 8 to 10 seconds.
5. Remove Aplicap and place in Applier. Raise the dispensing tip and pass to the dentist for placement. Pass a placement instrument.

COMPOSITE RESTORATION WITH TETRIC MICROHYBRID MATERIAL

This procedure is performed by the dentist and the dental assistant at chairside.

EQUIPMENT AND SUPPLIES:

- Basic set up
- Air/water syringe tip, HVE, and saliva ejector
- Cotton rolls and 2×2 gauze sponges, applicator tips
- Topical and local anesthetic setup
- Rubber dam setup
- High and low speed dental handpieces and assortment of diamond and cutting burs

- Spoon excavator
- Shade guide
- Plastic filling instrument
- Celluloid matrix strip and wedges
- Etchant and bonding agent or all in one etchant and bonding agent
- Plastic filling instrument (PFI)
- Tetic Microhybrid Composite Restorative System
- Curing light
- Finishing burs/diamonds, discs, and stones

DIRECTIONS:

1. Select the shade under natural light before the procedure begins. The tooth should be clean.
2. The anesthetic is given and the dental dam is placed for isolation.
3. The dentist prepares the cavity to receive the restoration material.

4. The dental assistant places a liner if required. Check composite instructions for type of material to select. Assistant mixes the material usually calcium hydroxide or glass ionomer liner and holds the pad, applicator, and a 2 × 2 gauze near the patients chin. After each application wipe the instrument. Light-cure if required.

5. Place the matrix and the wedge.

6. Place a dispensing tip on the etchant syringe and place the etchant for 10 to 20 seconds. Wash and rinse the tooth thoroughly for 20 to 30 seconds.

7. Using the air, gently remove any excess moisture.

8. Using a small application brush or cotton tipped applicator place the bonding agent, gently dry to remove any moisture and then light-cure approximately 10 seconds.
Note: An all in one etchant/bonding agent may also be used. This material is placed in one step. Refer to Chapter 1 Preliminary Restorative Materials for more information.

9. Prepare the selected shades of Tetric (Tetric comes in either Cavifils or the syringe.
10. Secure the Cavifils in the dispensing gun and then remove the tip or remove the cap from the Tetric syringe and dispense some material onto a paper pad. Pass to the dentist for placement.
11. Tetric is placed in increments and each increment is light-cured after placement for 40 seconds.
12. Several shades may be used to achieve the desired results of matching the tooth coloring.
13. Remove the wedge and matrix strip and pass an explorer to the dentist.
14. Rubber dam may be removed here, depends on dentist's preference.
15. Prepare and pass high speed hand piece with fine diamond and/or finishing burs to remove the excess material.
16. Pass finishing strip to finish the proximal surfaces.

17. Pass articulating forceps/paper to the dentist to check the occlusion.
18. Pass the low speed hand piece with silicone polishers, polishing discs, and polishing strips.
19. Rinse and evacuate.

MANUFACTURER:
Dentsply Caulk

USE:
- Making dental impressions used for the fabrication of casts for:
  - Study models
  - Orthodontic models
  - Opposing models
  - Removable splints
  - Removable retainers
  - Provisional restorations
  - Additional applications in the dental office

COMPOSITION:
- Crystaline Silica
- Amorphous Silica
- Calcium Sulfate

- Tetrasodium Pyrophosphate
- Potassium Alginate
- Magnesium Oxide
- Organic Glycol
- D & C Red #30 (Fast Set)
- Yellow Iron Oxide (Regular Set)

PROPERTIES:

- Supplied in airtight pouches or can (canister), water measure, and a scoop
- Material is supplied with a scoop and measuring device
- Appears to be a creamy color when mixed
- Comes in regular and fast set

OSHA PRECAUTIONS:

- Always read the MSDS information on the product
- Eye contact
- Inhalation

- Ingestion
- Patients who have history of severe allergic reactions to components

MIXING AND SETTING TIME:

	Regular Set	Fast Set
Mixing time	1 minute	45 seconds
Total working time	2:15 min/sec	1:30 min/sec
Initial setting time	2:30 min/sec	1:45 min/sec
Setting time	3:30 min/sec	2:30 min/sec

*The temperature of the water will vary the working and setting time. Cooler water increases time; warmer water decreases time.

DIRECTIONS:

After the tray is selected, PPE in place, and the patient is prepared for procedure:

1. Cut pouch and place into canister with tight-fitting lid
2. Fluff powder with lid in place

3. Dispense material by dipping supplied scoop into powder (do not pack) and tap it lightly against the rim to ensure that the scoop is filled. Use spatula by laying it level across the scoop to scrape excess material from the scoop.

4. Place scoops into dry mixing bowl (rubber bowl), disposable bowl, or into alginate mixer). Place additional scoops into bowl. Normally two scoops are needed for the mandibular and three scoops for the maxillary arch.

5. Add water from the water measuring device. Each line indicates enough water for one scoop. If three scoops are used, the entire water measuring device can be used. Water should be distilled and the water temperature should be approximately 73°F or 23°C.

6. Use a wide blade spatula to mix water and powder carefully at first to incorporate it together. Then spatulate against the bowl sides to reduce air incorporations. Do not whip the material. Rotate the bowl and gather the material and then spatulate again

against the sides of the bowl. Follow the mixing times for the material.

7. Once the material is mixed to a creamy texture without air bubbles, it can be gathered and loaded into the impression tray for insertion into the mouth.

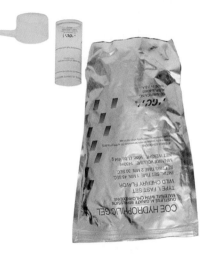

COE HYDROPHILIC GEL

DUSTLESS ALGINATE IMPRESSION
MATERIAL WITH CHLORHEXIDINE

TYPE I, FAST SET
WILD CHERRY FLAVOR

INITIAL SET TIME 1 MIN, 45 SEC.
SETTING TIME 2 MIN, 30 SEC.
MIN./MAX. VOLUME 1450ML
NET WEIGHT: 16oz. (1.0) 454 g

GC AMERICA INC.
MADE IN U.S.A.

MANUFACTURER:
GC America

USE:
Making dental impressions used for the fabrication of casts for:
- Study models
- Orthodontic models
- Opposing models
- Removable splints
- Removable retainers
- Provisional restorations
- Additional applications in the dental office

PROPERTIES:
- Supplied in airtight Ziplock® pouches with a water measure and a scoop
- Use scoop and water measure that is supplied with the material
- Low flow minimizes gagging
- High compressive strength

- High tear strength
- Comes in regular and fast set in both mint and cherry flavors

OSHA PRECAUTIONS:

- Always read the MSDS information on the product
- Eye contact
- Inhalation
- Ingestion
- Patients who have history of severe allergic reactions to components

MIXING AND SETTING TIME:

	Regular Set	Fast Set
Mixing time	45 seconds	45 seconds
Total working time	2:35 min/sec	1:35 min/sec
Initial setting time	2:50 min/sec	1:50 min/sec
Setting time	3:45 min/sec	2:45 min/sec

*The temperature of the water will vary the working and setting time. Cooler water increases time; warmer water decreases time.

DIRECTIONS:

After the tray is selected, PPE in place, and the patient is prepared for procedure:

1. Dispense material by dipping supplied scoop into powder and packing it into the scoop. Use spatula by laying it level across the scoop to further pack the material and scrape excess material from the scoop.

2. Place scoops into dry mixing bowl (rubber bowl, disposable bowl, or into alginate mixer). Place additional scoops into bowl. Normally two scoops are needed for the mandibular and three scoops for the maxillary arch.

3. Add water from the water measuring device. Each line indicates enough water for one scoop. If three scoops are used, the entire water measuring device can be used. Water should be distilled and at approx. 73°F or 23°C.

4. Use a wide blade spatula to mix water and powder carefully at first to incorporate it together. Then spatulate against the bowl sides to reduce air incorporations. Do not whip the material. Rotate the bowl and gather the material and then spatulate again against the sides of the bowl. Follow the mixing times for the material.

5. Once the material is mixed to a creamy texture without air bubbles, it can be gathered and loaded into the impression tray for insertion into the mouth.

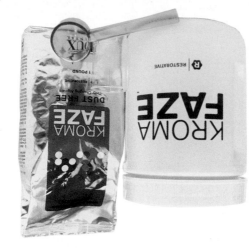

KROMAFAZE ALGINATE

MANUFACTURER:
DUX Dental

USE:
- Making dental impressions used for the fabrication of casts for:
  - Study models
  - Orthodontic models
  - Opposing models
  - Removable splints
  - Removable retainers
  - Provisional restorations
  - Additional applications in the dental office

PROPERTIES:
- Supplied in airtight pouches, with a water measure and a scoop
- Use scoop and water measure that is supplied with material

- High compressive strength
- High tear strength
- Stone models can be separated after 30 minutes
- Dust free
- Color changing guide for consistency
- Comes in regular and fast set

OSHA PRECAUTIONS:

- Always read the MSDS information on the product
- Eye contact
- Inhalation
- Ingestion
- Patients who have history of severe allergic reactions to components

MIXING AND SETTING TIME:
Visual color changing guide for consistency

	Regular	Fast
Mix	Purple	Purple
Load	Pink	Pink
Seat	White	White
Set		30–45 seconds

*The temperature of the water will vary the working and setting time. Cooler water increases time; warmer water decreases time.

DIRECTIONS:
After the tray is selected, PPE in place, and the patient is prepared for procedure:

1. Dispense material by dipping supplied scoop into powder and packing it into the scoop. Use spatula by laying it level across the scoop to further pack the material and scrape excess material from the scoop.

2. Place scoops into dry mixing bowl (rubber bowl), disposable bowl, or into alginate mixer). Place additional scoops into bowl. Normally two scoops are needed for the mandibular and three scoops for the maxillary arch.

3. Add water from the water measuring device. Each line indicates enough water for one scoop. If three scoops are used, the entire water measuring device can be used.

4. Use a wide blade spatula to mix water and powder carefully at first to incorporate it together. Then spatulate against the bowl sides to reduce air incorporations. Do not whip the material. Spatulate until the material turns to a pink color. Rotate the bowl and gather the material and then spatulate again against the sides of the bowl. Mix to a creamy consistency where all the powder is incorporated. Load the pink material into the tray.

5. When the material turns from pink to white, seat the tray into the patient's mouth and wait until the material is firm to remove.

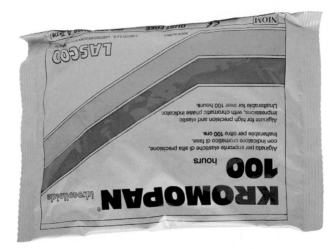

KROMOPAN® 100 ALGINATE

MANUFACTURER:
Kromopan USA, Inc.

USE:
- Making dental impressions used for the fabrication of casts for:
  - Study models
  - Orthodontic models
  - Opposing models
  - Removable splints
  - Removable retainers
  - Provisional restorations
  - When impression cannot be poured immediately
  - Additional applications in the dental office

PROPERTIES:
- Supplied in airtight pouches, with a water measure and a scoop
- Use scoop and water measure that is supplied with material
- Great elasticity

- High compression resistance
- Can be kept for up to 100 hours without distortion or shrinkage before pouring
- Color changing guide for consistency

OSHA PRECAUTIONS:

- Always read the MSDS information on the product
- Eye contact
- Inhalation
- Ingestion
- Patients who have history of severe allergic reactions to components

MIXING AND SETTING TIME:

Visual color changing guide for consistency

Spatulate	Purple
Load Tray	Pink
Insert into mouth	White

Time from start to finish is just over 1 minute.

*The temperature of the water will vary the working and setting time. Cooler water increases time; warmer water decreases time.

DIRECTIONS:

After the tray is selected, PPE in place, and the patient is prepared for procedure:

1. Dispense material by dipping supplied scoop into powder and packing it into the scoop. Use spatula by laying it level across the scoop to further pack the material and scrape excess material from the scoop.
2. Place scoops into dry mixing bowl (rubber bowl, disposable bowl, or into alginate mixer). Place additional scoops into the bowl. Normally two scoops are needed for the mandibular and three scoops for the maxillary arch.
3. Add water from the water measuring device. Each line indicates enough water for one scoop. If three scoops are used, the entire water measuring device can be used.

4. Use a wide blade spatula to mix water and powder carefully at first to incorporate it together. Then spatulate against the bowl sides to reduce air incorporations. Do not whip the material. Spatulate until the material turns to a pink color. Rotate the bowl and gather the material and then spatulate again against the sides of the bowl. Mix to a creamy consistency where all the powder is incorporated. Load the pink material into the tray.

5. When the material turns from pink to white, seat the tray into the patient's mouth and wait until the material is firm to remove. After removal the impression can be rinsed and enclosed in a plastic bag and kept without distortion for up to 100 hours.

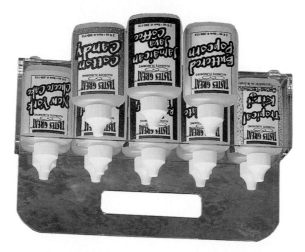

ALGINATE FLAVORING

MANUFACTURER:
Ortho Technology, Inc.

USE:
To add a pleasing flavor to alginate products

PROPERTIES:
- Supplied in 2 oz. dropper bottles
- 10–14 sugar-free flavors
- Alginate Flavoring Carrier is available for use with 10 different flavors
- Flavors available:
  - Very Strawberry
  - Marvelous Mint
  - Chillin'Cherry
  - Groovy Grape
  - Wild Watermelon
  - Bubble Gum

- Georgia Peach
- Cotton Candy
- French Vanilla
- Orange Dreamsicle
- Buttered Popcorn
- Jamaican Java Coffee
- New York Cheesecake
- Tropical Kiwi

OSHA PRECAUTIONS:

- Patients who have history of severe allergic reactions to components

DIRECTIONS:

1. Patients identify alginate flavoring preference
2. Plastic barrier is placed around dropper bottle
3. Operator adds 2 to 5 drops in water before mixing it with the alginate powder

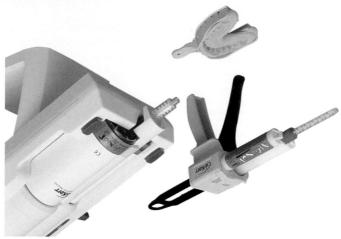

ALGINOT™

MANUFACTURER:
Kerr Corporation

USE:
- For impressions in preparation of:
  - Case study models
  - Orthodontic models
  - Opposing models
  - Simple removable dentures
  - Removable retainers and splints
  - Provisional crown and bridge

COMPOSITION:
- A silicone impression material intended as an alternative to traditional alginate materials

PROPERTIES:
- Extruder operation with mixing tip and cartridge—no hand mixing
- Impressions remain stable for months
- Tolerates disinfectants

OSHA PRECAUTIONS:

- Skin, eyes: may cause mild irritation
- Inhalation: may cause mild irritation
- May be harmful if swallowed

MIXING AND SETTING TIME:

	Minimum Working Time from Start of Mix	Removal Time
Cartridge:	0:45 minute	2:30 minutes
Volume™	1:00 minute	2:45 minutes

DIRECTIONS:

After the tray is selected, PPE in place, and the patient is prepared for procedure:

1. Insert cartridge into the extruder.
2. Attach mixing tip to cartridge.
3. Squeeze trigger to mix and dispense material.
4. Material will stop flowing when trigger is released.

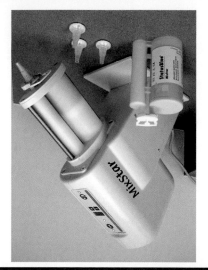

STATUSBLUE ® MIX STAR MATERIAL
(ALGINATE SUBSTITUTE MATERIAL)

MANUFACTURER:
Zenith/DMG

USE:
- Making dental impressions used for the fabrication of casts for:
  - Study models
  - Orthodontic models
  - Opposing models
  - Impressions for temporaries
  - Model-cast dentures
  - Additional applications in the dental office

COMPOSITION:
- Addition curing polysiloxanes
- Silicon dioxide
- Food pigments
- Additives
- Platinum catalyst

PROPERTIES:

- Designed at a high efficiency alternative to traditional alginates
- Supplied automix cartridges for use with a Zenith/DMG MixStar machine
- Automix Gun Tips are used with the automix cartridges
- StatusBlue® also supplied in 50 ml cartridges for automix guns and tips
- 100% dust-free
- Mixing takes place in the MixStar machine if using the MixStar cartridges
- Extremely flowable under pressure
- Low shore hardness
- Dimensionally stable
- Repourable and reusable
- StatusBlue is an additional curing silicone impression material

OSHA PRECAUTIONS:

- Always read the MSDS information on the product

- On MSDS: under Hazards Identification it reads: "None if handled according to directions." "No labeling of hazardous ingredients required."
- Patients who have history of severe allergic reactions to components

MIXING AND SETTING TIME:

Tray is loaded and inserted into mouth no later than	1:15 after mixing
Recommended Time in Mouth	1:45 minutes

*Must wait a minimum of 30 minutes before pouring impression

DIRECTIONS:

1. Slide the locking mechanism into open position on the MixStar Cartridge.
2. Remove and discard the cap on the openings of the base and catalyst outlets on the MixStar Cartridge.
3. Seat the mixing tip completely into the open holes on the MixStar Cartridge.

4. Secure the mixing tip by sliding the locking mechanism into locked position over the mixing tip.
5. Insert the cartridge into the mixing unit.
6. Turn on the mixing unit and as the material is dispensed flow the material into the tray keeping the tip in the material and not trapping air into the material.
7. Insert the tray into the patient's mouth and hold for 1:45 minutes
8. Remove from the patient's mouth, rinse, and disinfect.
9. Wait 30 minutes and pour the impression.

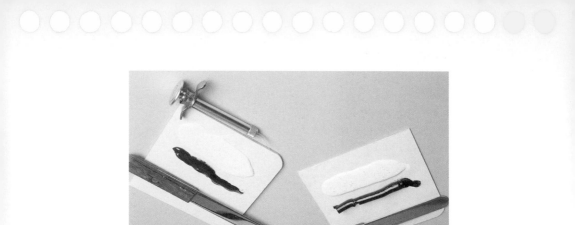

MANUFACTURER:
GC America

USE:
- For taking impressions for the following:
  - Full dentures
  - Partial dentures
  - Inlays
  - Onlays
  - Crowns
  - Bridges

PROPERTIES:
- Lead-free
- High elasticity
- Excellent tear strength
- Blue-green color, mint flavor
- Available in 3 viscosities
- Three-year shelf life

- Available in Regular Body, Injection Type (Light), Heavy Body, and Fast Set
- Unmixed catalyst or base may stain clothes

OSHA PRECAUTIONS:

- Always read the MSDS information on the product
- MSDS indications refer to the accelerator
- Disposable vinyl gloves recommended
- Eye protection
- Respirator protection
- Ventilation

MIXING AND SETTING TIME:

	Light-bodied	Medium-bodied	Medium-bodied	Heavy bodied
Material Type	Type 3	Type 2	Fast Set-Type 2	Type 1
Mixing time	45 sec–1 min	45 sec–1 min	30 sec	45 sec–1 min
Min. time in mouth	8–10 min	8–10 min	4 min	8–10 min

*To speed up setting time, use more catalyst; to retard setting time, use less catalyst.

DIRECTIONS:

After the tray is selected, PPE in place, and the patient is prepared for procedure:

1. Paint the entire surface of the tray with the tray adhesive. When dry, begin mixing the catalyst and base.
2. The catalyst and base are dispensed by using equal lengths. This is about one part catalyst to two parts base according to volume. The diameter of the dispensed material should be the same diameter as the orifice of the tubes.
3. Coat the spatula with the blue paste before incorporating the blue and white pastes together. Spatulate with broad strokes until it is free from streaks.
4. Fill an impression syringe with material (injection type—light) to inject onto and around the preparation.
5. Fill the impression tray that has been painted with adhesive with material (regular body or heavy body).

6. Firmly place into the oral cavity. Do not apply pressure against the tray while the material is setting. Do not remove impression prematurely. Hold in place for the minimum time indicated. With a blunt instrument, check material for setting prior to removal.

7. Break seal with lateral movement and remove impression with a straight pull. Rinse off and disinfect or sterilize.

8. Pour model no later than 8 hours.

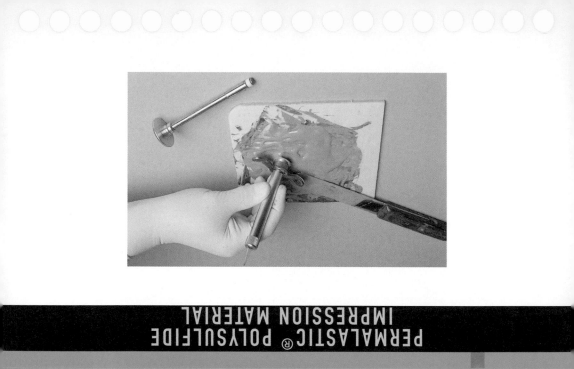

MANUFACTURER:
Kerr Corporation

USE:
- Regular is recommended for partial or full denture impressions.
- Light is for inlay and fixed bridge impressions.

PROPERTIES:
- Has a high degree of flow
- Good tear strength
- Comes in Regular, Light-Bodied, and Heavy-Bodied
- An adhesive is available in a 2 oz. size.

OSHA PRECAUTIONS:
- Always read the MSDS information on the product.
- Use safety glasses and gloves.
- Use protective clothing because this product may cause staining.
- This material may cause irritation to skin and eyes.

- If ingested, this material may cause choking sensation.
- This product contains a lead compound.

MIXING AND SETTING TIME:

Mixing time	.75–1.0 minute
Tray loading	1.0 minute
Syringe filling	10.0 min. from start of mix
Mouth removal	6 min. in mouth

DIRECTIONS:

After the tray is selected, PPE in place, and the patient is prepared for procedure:

1. Extrude appropriate amounts of base and catalyst pastes onto a mixing pad. Use equal lengths not equal amounts.
2. Using a laboratory spatula, mix materials into each other using a stirring motion.
3. Incorporate thoroughly until a streak-free mix is obtained.
4. Mixing should be completed within 45 seconds to 1 minute.

5. Immediately fill tray or syringe.
6. The material must stay in the mouth for a minimum of 6 minutes.
7. Remove and disinfect by immersion in a 2% solution of gluteraldehyde.
8. Pouring should occur immediately or within 8 hours.

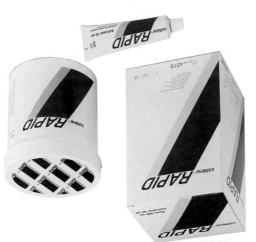

COLTENE® RAPID IMPRESSION MATERIAL

MANUFACTURER:
Coltene/Whaledent, Inc.

USE:
- For inlay and fixed bridge impressions
- Partial and full denture impressions

PROPERTIES:
- Condensation silicone impression material
- Seven-day dimensional stability
- Material changes color during mixing for easy and reliable handling
- Surface-activated hydrophilic to enhance performance when in contact with moist oral tissue
- It is available in putty, liner with activators and applicator.
- Dosing spoon and dosing syringe are available as well.

MIXING AND SETTING TIME:

Mixing time   30 seconds
Oral setting time   150 seconds

DIRECTIONS:

After the tray is selected, PPE in place, and the patient is prepared for procedure:

1. Measure the required quantity of Rapid line base into the applicator.
2. Add red activator with the precision syringe.
3. Stir briefly. The material turns blue when it's ready for use.
4. Rapid liner is applied from the applicator directly into the primary impression tray or into the syringe.
5. Place into the oral cavity and remove when set.

Courtesy of 3M ESPE

IMPREGUM™ PENTA™ POLYETHER
IMPRESSION MATERIAL

MANUFACTURER:
3M ESPE

USE:
- Impressions of inlay, onlay, veneer, crown, and bridge preparations
- Fixation and implant impressions

PROPERTIES:
- Comes in tubes, Penta cartridges, syringe in medium and soft medium body
- Intrinsic pre-setting hydrophilicity helps capture and reproduce outstanding detail.

OSHA PRECAUTIONS:
- Face and eye protection
- Do not ingest.
- Avoid prolonged or repeated skin contact.

MIXING AND SETTING TIME:

Processing time from start of mixing	1:00 minute max
Residence time in the mouth	3:00 minutes
Setting time from start of mixing	4:00 minute max

DIRECTIONS:

After the tray is selected, PPE in place, and the patient is prepared for procedure:

1. The dosing and mixing are done automatically in the Pentamix 2.
2. If using the tubes, dispense in equal lengths and mix until streak-free.

POLYJEL® NF™ POLYETHER IMPRESSION MATERIAL

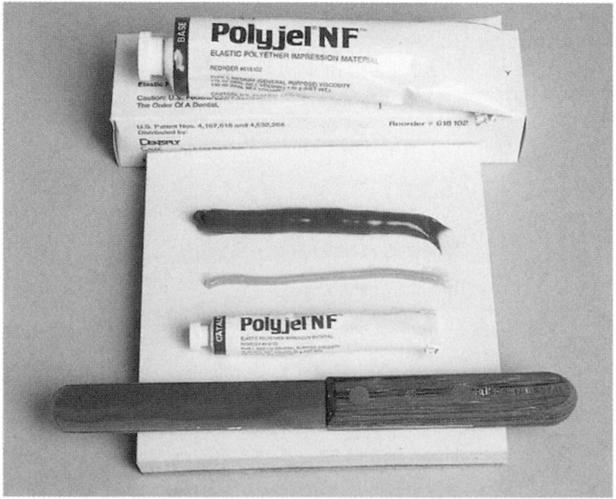

MANUFACTURER:
Dentsply Caulk

USE:
- Reproduction for crown and bridge impressions

PROPERTIES:
- Easy-to-release polyether-type elastomeric impression material
- Single viscosity that provides optimum performance
- Dimensional stability
- Fast set time

OSHA PRECAUTIONS:
- Always read the MSDS information on the product.
- Base paste and catalyst paste
- Avoid eye and skin contact and ingestion.
- Protective eyeglasses to be worn
- Protective rubber gloves to be worn

- Rubber apron for protective clothing
- Do not eat, drink, or smoke when using.

MIXING AND SETTING TIME:

Mix material	30–45 seconds
Total working time	2.5 minutes

DIRECTIONS:

After the tray is selected, PPE in place, and the patient is prepared for procedure:

1. Measure the required quantity of PolyJel base and catalyst onto mixing pad.
2. The material is dispensed in equal lengths not equal amounts within 45 seconds.
3. Spatulate with broad blade spatula and mix until streak–free.
4. Place into the oral cavity and remove when set.
5. Material must be poured within 2 weeks.

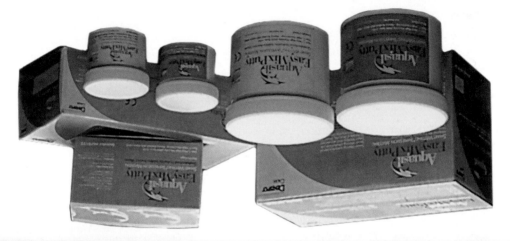

AQUASIL SMART WETTING® VINYL POLYSILOXANE
IMPRESSION MATERIAL

MANUFACTURER:
Dentsply Caulk

USE:
- Suitable for all impression techniques where high viscosity materials would be desired by the operator
- This material can be used for duplication of models.

COMPOSITION:
- Aquasil Putty Impression Material is a quadrafunctional hydrophilic addition reaction silicone.

PROPERTIES:
- Designed to minimize the problems of voids, bubbles, pulls, and drags
- Wetability
- High tear strength
- Available in broad range, many viscosities in regular and fast set
- Mint-flavored

OSHA PRECAUTIONS:

- Always read the MSDS information on the product.
- Use safety glasses and gloves.
- Avoid eye and skin contact and ingestion.

MIXING AND SETTING TIME:

	Regular	Fast Set
Working time	2:15–2:45 min	1:15–1:45 min
Setting time from start of mix	5:00 min	3:00 min

DIRECTIONS:

After the tray is selected, PPE in place, and the patient is prepared for procedure:

1. Insert the cartridge into the extruder.
2. Attach the mixing tip to the cartridge.
3. Squeeze the trigger to mix and dispense material.
4. Material will stop flowing when the trigger is released.

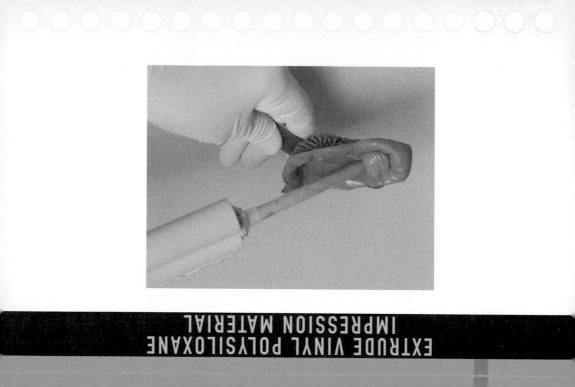

EXTRUDE VINYL POLYSILOXANE
IMPRESSION MATERIAL

MANUFACTURER:
Kerr Corporation

USE:
- It is suitable for all crown and bridge, edentulous and implant impressions.

PROPERTIES:
- Thixotropic, non-slumping tray material
- Available in cartridge, putty (jars), and tube
- High flow and tear strength
- Putty has 3-year shelf life
- Dimensional stability
- Tasteless
- Odorless

OSHA PRECAUTIONS:
- May cause mild skin irritation
- May cause irritation to the eyes
- May be harmful if swallowed
- May cause mild irritation if inhaled

MIXING AND SETTING TIME:

	Total Working Time from start of mix	Minimum Removal Time from start of mix
Extrude Wash	3:00 min	6:00 min
Extrude Medium	3:00 min	6:00 min
Extrude Extra	3:00 min	6:00 min
Extrude MPV	2:15 min	5:15 min
Extrude Putty	2:00 min	6:00 min

DIRECTIONS:

After the tray is selected, PPE in place, and the patient is prepared for procedure:

1. Insert the cartridge into the extruder.
2. Attach the mixing tip to the cartridge.
3. Squeeze the trigger to mix and dispense material.
4. The material will stop flowing when the trigger is released.

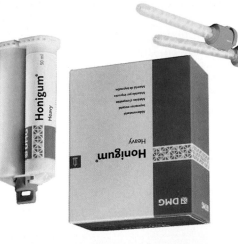

HONIGUM® IMPRESSION MATERIAL

MANUFACTURER:
Zenith/DMG

USE:
- Crown and bridge impressions
- Inlay and onlay impressions
- All types of pickup impression, e.g., for implants

COMPOSITION:
- Addition curing polysiloxanes, silicone dioxide, food pigments, additives, and platinum catalyst

PROPERTIES:
- Patented microcrystalline wax matrix chemistry
- Pressure-sensitive variable viscosity
- Mild honey aroma for great patient acceptance

MANUFACTURER:
Zenith/DMG

USE:
- Crown and bridge impressions
- Inlay and onlay impressions
- All types of pickup impression, e.g., for implants

COMPOSITION:
- Addition curing polysiloxanes, silicone dioxide, food pigments, additives, and platinum catalyst

PROPERTIES:
- Patented microcrystalline wax matrix chemistry
- Pressure-sensitive variable viscosity
- Mild honey aroma for great patient acceptance

OSHA PRECAUTIONS:

- Hand and skin protection: use rubber gloves.
- Eye protection: use goggles.
- Consult a physician in case of ingestion.

MIXING AND SETTING TIME:

	Automix Heavy	Automix Heavy Fast	MixStar Heavy	MixStar Heavy Fast
Working time	2:00 min	1:15 min	2:15 min	1:15 min
Recommended time in mouth	3:15 min	2:00 min	3:15 min	2:00 min

DIRECTIONS:

After the tray is selected, PPE in place, and the patient is prepared for procedure:

1. Slide the locking mechanism into open position on the MixStar cartridge.
2. Remove and discard the cap on the openings of the base and catalyst outlets on the MixStar cartridge.

3. Seat the mixing tip completely into the open holes on the MixStar cartridge.
4. Secure the mixing tip by sliding the locking mechanism into locked position over the mixing tip.
5. Insert the cartridge into the mixing unit.
6. Turn on the mixing unit and as the material is dispensed, flow the material into the tray keeping the tip in the material and not trapping air into the material.
7. Insert the tray into the patient's mouth and hold time noted according to material used.
8. Remove from patient's mouth, rinse, and disinfect.
9. Wait 30 minutes and pour the impression.

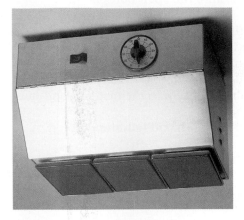

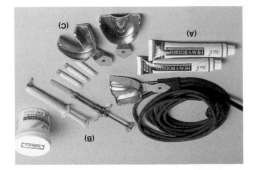

HYDROCOLLOID-REVERSIBLE HYDROCOLLOID
IMPRESSION MATERIAL

MANUFACTURER:

Van R

USE:

- Crown and bridge impressions
- Inlay and onlay impressions

COMPOSITION:

- Made from water and the ocean's agar

PROPERTIES:

- Wetness
- Small amounts of blood and saliva do not affect the accuracy of the impression.
- Available in syringe and tubes
- Must be used with a Hydrocolloid machine

OSHA PRECAUTIONS:

- Principal hazardous components—none
- No occupational control measures needed

MIXING AND SETTING TIME:

Acculoid, Lavender, Extra Strength
5 minute temper at 110°F/43°C
7 minute cooling in the mouth with room temperature water
Stores 5 days once liquefied

Agarloid, Blue, Fast Tempering
4 minute temper at 110°F/43°C
5 minute cooling in the mouth with room temperature water
Stores 5 days once liquefied

Slate, Gray, High Strength
5 minute temper at 110°F/43°C
5 minute cooling in the mouth with room temperature water
Stores 4 days once liquefied

Qwik, Chocolate
  3 minute temper at 110°F/43°C
  3 minute cooling in the mouth with room temperature water
  Stores 3 days once liquefied

DIRECTIONS:

After the tray is selected, PPE in place, and the patient is prepared for procedure:

1. Remove the tube from the storage compartment of the hydrocolloid conditioner. Fill the water-cooled tray and place in the tempering bath.
2. Set the timer to the correct time for tempering according to the material being used.
3. After the time has concluded, remove the syringe material that is in the cartiloid and place it into the syringe. Attach a hydrocolloid syringe tip to the cartiloid and apply pressure to the syringe to expel a small amount of material while taking to

the operator to use. This ensures that the material does not set up in the tip.
4. Remove the impression from the tempering bath and place a 2 × 2 over the material to dry off the top surface. Attach the tubing to the impression and hand it to the operator to place into the mouth.
5. After the impression is seated in the mouth, attach the tubing to the water source and start the water flowing. Set the timer.
6. Remove from patient's mouth, rinse and pour immediately.

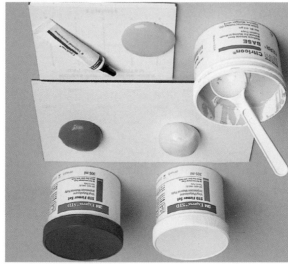

PROCEDURE: PREPARING A PRELIMINARY PUTTY IMPRESSION FROM A POLYSILOXANE IMPRESSION MATERIAL

1. Follow the manufacturer's directions.
2. Wear vinyl gloves.
3. Either equal scoops of the putty are mixed together or putty base and drops of catalyst are mixed together. The putty must be kneaded together until a homogeneous mixture is obtained within the manufacturer's recommended time. Normally, this time is 30 seconds. The mixture must be one even color with no streaks.
4. After the material is mixed, pat it into a patty and load it into the prepared tray. With a finger, make a slight indentation where the teeth are located.

5. Place the plastic spacer sheet over the material and insert it into the patient's mouth. The objective is to create 2 mm of space for the final syringeable viscous impression material.

6. The setting of the putty takes about 3 minutes. The tray is then removed from the patient's mouth, the spacer is removed, and the putty is checked for accuracy and left to set further.

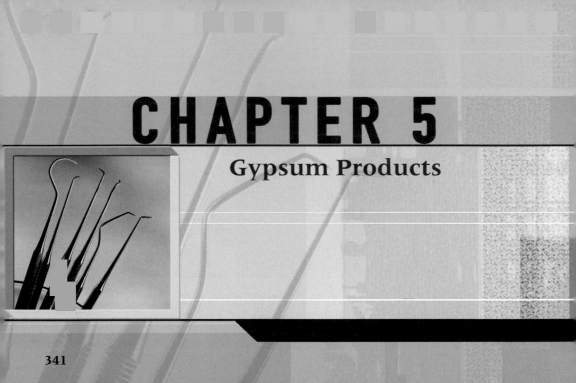

CHAPTER 5

Gypsum Products

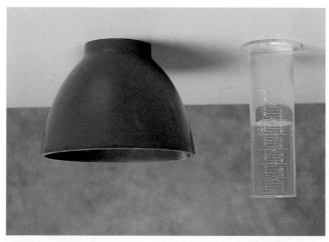

MANUFACTURER:
Pascal Company, Inc.

USE:
- Indicated for adults and children over 6 years of age
- For patients with recurrent decay around restorations and for those at risk for root caries
- Good for xerostomia-induced caries, orthodontic decalcification, and hypersensitivity

COMPOSITION:
- 1.1% sodium fluoride
- Sodium saccharin

PROPERTIES:
- Safe for porcelain crowns, bridges, or composite restorations
- Can be used in place of toothpaste
- Mild dentifrice cleaning that removes plaque
- Leaves mouth feeling fresh

- Highest level of fluoride allowed for take-home fluoride products
- Easy dispensing
- Nonallergenic and nonstaining
- Sodium benzoate free

OSHA PRECAUTIONS:

- May cause irritation to the eyes—flush for 15 minutes
- May cause irritation to the skin—wash for 15 minutes
- Ingestion: may cause nausea, vomiting, diarrhea, abdominal distress, and weakness—seek medical assistance if more than used for brushing is swallowed

MIXING AND SETTING TIME:

- No mixing required
- Leave gel on teeth for 1 minute

DIRECTIONS:

1. Adults and children 6 years or older use once a day at bedtime.

2. Brush and floss and then remove excess water from the toothbrush.
3. Liberally cover bristles of toothbrush with NeutraGard Advanced 1.1% Neutral Sodium Fluoride Gel.
4. Brush on to all tooth surfaces for 1 minute.
5. Do not swallow any material and do not rinse.
6. Expectorate thoroughly; do not rinse, eat, or drink for 30 minutes.
7. Children 6 years and older: Expectorate and rinse thoroughly.

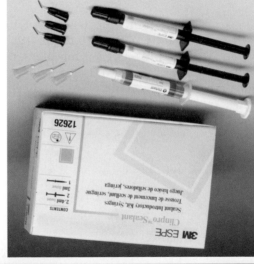

MANUFACTURER:
3M-ESPE Dental Products

USE:
- Sealing the enamel pits and fissures to protect against dental caries

COMPOSITION:
- Triethylene glycol dimethacrylate
- Bisphenol A diglycidyl ether dimethacrylate
- Tetrabutylammonium, tetrafluoroborate
- Silane-treated silica

PROPERTIES:
- Low viscosity
- Bonds to enamel
- Fluoride releasing
- Flows easily into pits and fissures

- Comes with ultra fine tips for easy placement
- Color change technology

OSHA PRECAUTIONS:

- May cause mild eye irritation
- May cause allergy to skin or moderate skin irritation
- Prolonged or repeated exposure may cause upper respiratory irritation
- May cause gastrointestinal irritation

MIXING AND SETTING TIME:

- No mixing required
- Sealant is light-cured for 20 seconds to set.

DIRECTIONS:

1. Prepare delivery system. Remove cap from the syringe and save.
2. Twist disposable cap onto the syringe until secure.
3. Dispense a small amount of material on a paper pad to ensure the tip is not clogged.

4. Etch each tooth according to the manufacturer's directions, then rinse thoroughly and air-dry. The tooth should be a matte frosty white color on the etched area.
5. Do not allow the etched surface to be contaminated.
6. Using the syringe tip, slowly introduce the pit and fissure sealant to the etched surface of the tooth.
7. Stirring the sealant during and after placement with the syringe tip or an explorer will help to eliminate air bubbles and enhance the flow of the sealant into the pits and fissures.
8. Hold the tip of the curing light close to the surface and cure for 20 seconds.
9. When set, the sealant forms a hard, opaque film that is light yellow in color with a slight inhibition.
10. Repeat this on each etched tooth.

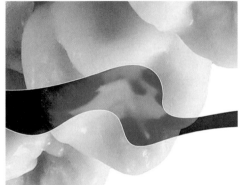

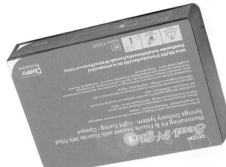

DELTON SEAL-N-GLO LIGHT CURE
PIT & FISSURE SEALANT

MANUFACTURER:
Dentsply Professional

USE:
- Preventive sealing of pits and fissures in the primary and secondary dentition in combination with the acid-etch techniques

COMPOSITION:
- Low viscosity monomers, triethylene glycol dimethacrylate, BisGMA, barium alumino fluroboro silicate glass, titanium dioxide, silicon dioxide, sodium fluoride, initiators, stabilizers, fluorescent dye—38% filled

PROPERTIES:
- Provides visual verification of sealant margins at time of placement
- Easy way to verify retention and integrity of margins at recall appointments

- Contains fluoride
- Effective sealing properties
- Illuminating dye does not color or change the look of the opaque sealant
- Easy to place

OSHA PRECAUTIONS:
- May cause eye irritation
- Individuals sensitive to acrylics may develop an allergic response.
- Possible nausea on prolonged exposure
- Possible irritation to the skin

MIXING AND SETTING TIME:
- No mixing required
- Setting: Light-cure to set

DIRECTIONS:
1. Tooth must be cleaned with an air polishing device or prophylaxis treatment.

2. Rinse well with water and isolate the teeth to be sealed.
3. Air-dry each tooth with air free of oil or water contamination.
4. Etch the pits and fissures of the teeth to be sealed for 15–60 seconds according to the manufacturer's directions.
5. Rinse thoroughly for at least 30 seconds, then dry area.
6. Teeth will have a dull frosty white appearance; if they do not look like this, re-etch for another 20 seconds.
7. Remove cap from the Delton Seal-N-Glo syringe. Attach a disposable applicator tip to end of the syringe. Turn the tip clockwise to secure the applicator tip to the end of the syringe.
8. Express a small amount onto a pad to assure free flow of material.
9. Apply the sealant into the pits and fissures.
10. Cure each surface for at least 20 seconds, keeping the curing light tip as close to the tooth surface without actually touching the tooth as possible.
11. Remove the soft (oxygen-inhibited) surface layer after light-curing with cotton pellets or cotton rolls.

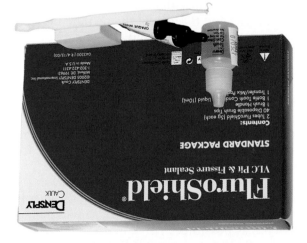

FLUROSHIELD VLC PIT & FISSURE SEALANT

MANUFACTURER:
Dentsply Caulk

USE:
- Preventive sealing in pits and fissures in primary and secondary dentition to protect against dental caries
- Fluoride release that is intended to act as a fluoride supplement

COMPOSITION:
- Urethane-modified Bis-GMA dimethacrylate
- Barium alumino fluroboro silicate glass
- Polymerizable dimethacrylate resins
- Bis-GMA
- Sodium fluoride
- Photoiniator
- Photoaccelerator
- Silicon dioxide
- 50% inorganic filler

PROPERTIES:

- Visible light-cured pit and fissure sealant
- Releasable fluoride that is intended to act as a fluoride supplement
- Decreases the chance of microleakage
- Bonds chemically and mechanically to the enamel
- Low water absorption increases resistance to washout

OSHA PRECAUTIONS:

- Material may cause irritation to the eyes.
- Material may be an irritant.
- Material is probably not harmful if swallowed.

MIXING AND SETTING TIME:

- No mixing is required.
- Material is light-cured for 20 seconds per surface.

DIRECTIONS:

1. Prophy the pits and fissures of the teeth to be sealed then rinse thoroughly and air–dry.

2. Isolate the teeth with cotton rolls or a rubber dam.
3. Apply Caulk 50% Tooth Conditioner Liquid with the cotton tip applicator for 60 seconds to permanent teeth and 90 seconds for primary teeth then rinse thoroughly and air–dry.
4. Tooth should look frosty.
5. Remove the cap and place FluoroShield material on a paper pad. Cover to protect from the overhead light.
6. Pick up a liberal amount of material using the disposable brush and place on the tooth into the pits and fissures.
7. Light-cure all surfaces keeping the tip of the light about 1–2 mm away from the surface for 20 seconds (curing time depends on the light source).

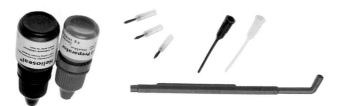

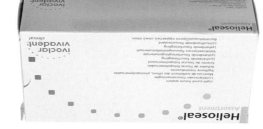

HELIOSEAL SEALANT

MANUFACTURER:
Ivoclar Vivadent

USE:
- Provides excellent long-term cavity protection in occlusal areas

COMPOSITION:
- Mixture of Bis-GMA, dimethacrylate, titanium dioxide, initiators, and stabilizers

PROPERTIES:
- Long-term caries protection
- Fast and easy to apply
- Has a white opaque shade
- Also available in three other formulas: A transparent sealer—Helioseal Clear; a transparent sealer with reversible color changes using a halogen polymerization light—Helioseal Clear Chroma; and a white-shaded sealant with additional fluoride release—Helioseal F

OSHA PRECAUTIONS:

- May be irritating to the eyes—flush with water
- Skin contact—wash thoroughly with soap and water
- Inhalation—move to fresh air
- No hazards anticipated with swallowing a small amount of material with normal handling

MIXING AND SETTING TIME:

- No mixing required
- 35 second total including waiting time and light-curing

DIRECTIONS:

1. Thoroughly clean the tooth to be sealed.
2. Isolate the area preferably with a rubber dam.
3. Place the disposable tip on Syringe Total Etch and apply the etching gel for 30–60 seconds, then thoroughly rinse and dry with oil-free air. Tooth should have a mat appearance.
4. Shake the Helioseal bottle well and open immediately before use to prevent any premature polymerization by light.

5. Remove the cap and place a cannula on the bottle to apply directly or place Helioseal in well, on paper pad, or directly dispense from bottle and apply with the brush handle and tip supplied in the kit.
6. Wait for 15 seconds and then light-cure with a suitable light source for 20 seconds.
7. Check seal and occlusion.

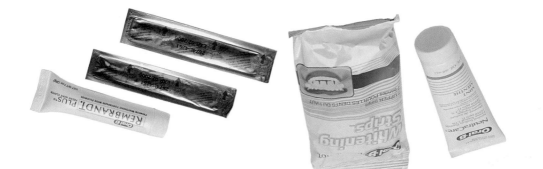

MANUFACTURER:
Rembrandt

USE:
- To whiten teeth
- To restore the original brightness of professional whitening

COMPOSITION:
- PVP, PEG8, water, acrylate copolymer, hydrogen peroxide, disodium pyrophosphate, sodium stannate, disodium EDTA

PROPERTIES:
- Noticeably whiter teeth in 5 days
- Only apply once a day compared to twice-daily with other systems
- Form fit strips
- Economical yet effective whitening
- Quick results and easy application
- Adheres well to the tooth

OSHA PRECAUTIONS:

- May cause irritation to the eyes
- May cause skin irritation and blanching
- If swallowed, contact your doctor immediately or the Poison Control Center.

MIXING AND SETTING TIMES:

- No mixing required

DIRECTIONS:

1. Rinse mouth with water for 15 seconds to moisten the teeth.
2. Remove the upper strip from the blister pack.
3. Apply the upper strip by aligning the straight edge with the gum line and pressing down to fit the curves of the teeth.
4. Press the tabs behind the front teeth to secure strip.
5. Remove the lower strip from the blister pack and repeat the same process on the lower teeth.
6. Wear the strips for 30 minutes and avoid eating, drinking, or smoking.

7. After 30 minutes, rinse mouth with water for 15 seconds.
8. Remove the strips from the upper and lower teeth. Discard the used strips.
9. If whiter teeth are desired, continue using the strips for 7 days.

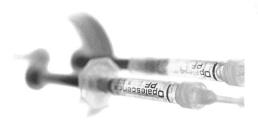

OPALESCENCE TOOTH WHITENING SYSTEMS

MANUFACTURER:
Ultradent Products, Inc.

USE:
- Whiten the teeth
- Removing the colors present on teeth from the time of tooth eruption and/or the stains of aging
- Success with varying degrees of tetracycline and brown fluorosis discoloration
- Used on nonvital teeth for intracoronal bleaching

COMPOSITION:
- Carbamide peroxide
- Potassium nitrate
- Fluoride ion

PROPERTIES:
- Very effective bleaching agent
- Comes in unit dose syringes and is flavored

- Available in different percentages of carbamide peroxide
- Has sustained release
- Adhesive properties
- Custom designed application tray
- High-viscosity and sticky

OSHA PRECAUTIONS:
- Eyes—immediately flush eyes for 15 minutes
- Skin—wash with soap and water thoroughly
- Ingestion—if swallowed, give the patient a glass of water or milk and call a physician.
- Inhalation—not defined

MIXING AND SETTING TIMES:
- No mixing is required.
- Application time varies depending on the patient's needs, level of sensitivity, and day-to-day activities.

DIRECTIONS:

1. Fabricate the tray according to the manufacturer's instructions.
2. Instruct the patient on the bleaching procedure.
3. Patient should load gel into their custom tray. Use 1/2 to 1 full syringe of material to fill the tray.
4. Brush the teeth, and then insert the tray. Adapt tray sides to the teeth.
5. Remove excess gel with a clean finger or soft toothbrush. Rinse twice; do not swallow rinses.
6. The dentist will instruct the patient when and how long to bleach. Opalescence carbamide peroxide gel will bleach 8–10 hours during the night or 4–6 hours during the day. In some treatment sequences the bleaching procedure is completed by the patient for 30 minutes several times a day.
7. Patient is evaluated every 3 to 5 days of treatment or as needed.

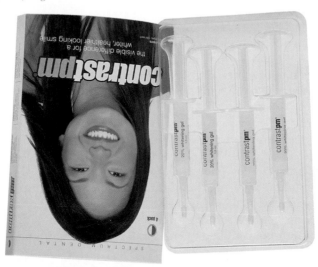

CONTRASTPM WHITENING SYSTEMS

MANUFACTURER:
Spectrum Dental

USE:
- Tooth whitening system

COMPOSITION:
- Propylene glycol, hydroxlpropyl, glycerin, spearmint oil, fumed silica, tetra potassium, pyrophosphate, carbamide peroxide, emulating wax, and hydrogen peroxide

PROPERTIES:
- Neutral pH
- Mild spearmint flavor
- Fast, effective whitening
- Cream texture, viscous gel material
- Offers extended contact and prolonged carbamide peroxide release
- Comes in different percentages

OSHA PRECAUTIONS:

- Eyes—immediately flush eyes for 15 minutes
- Skin—wash with soap and water thoroughly
- Ingestion—if ingested, may cause irritation; contact physician

MIXING AND SETTING TIMES:

- No mixing required
- Contact time depends on strength of solution and patient's level of sensitivity

DIRECTIONS:

1. Place a drop of ContrastPM whitening gel in the center of each tooth compartment of the custom fit tray.
2. Place the tray in the mouth and compress the gel against the tooth, dispersing the material across the surface.
3. Do not over-fill the trays, as the overflow may irritate the gingival tissues. Remove any excess with your finger or a dry toothbrush.
4. You may rinse gently for 5 seconds, if needed.

5. Follow the dentist's instruction, carefully regarding the treatment plan.
6. The 10% and 15% whitening gels can be worn in the trays overnight or during the day for up to 4 hours.
7. The 20% whitening gels can be worn for 1 hour and up to 2 hours if no sensitivity exists.
8. After the trays are removed, rinse and brush excess gel from the teeth. Rinse the trays with cold water using a toothbrush to remove any gel. Store trays in the case in a cool, dry place.

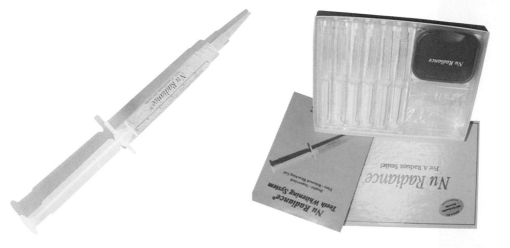

Courtesy of Nu Radiance, Inc.

NU RADIANCE DUET TOOTH WHITENING SYSTEM

MANUFACTURER:
Nu Radiance

USE:
- To whiten teeth without sensitivity

COMPOSITION:
- Stabilized carbamide peroxide gel mixed with an accelerator and hydrating agent

PROPERTIES:
- Easy, comfortable, and effective whitening system
- Takes less time
- Comes in different percentages
- Hydrates the teeth so it does not cause sensitivity

OSHA PRECAUTIONS:
- May cause irritation to the eyes—flush with copious amount of water

- May cause skin irritation—wash with soap and water
- If swallowed, drink large amounts of water and contact your doctor immediately
- No harm anticipated if inhaled in the amount of commercially packaged material

MIXING AND SETTING TIMES:
- No mixing is required.
- Application times vary with the percentage of solution.

DIRECTIONS:
1. Remove the tip guard and place a mixing tip securely on the syringe.
2. Do not pull back on the syringe as this may activate the gel.
3. Pat the teeth dry before treatment.
4. Place a small line of gel on the front of the tray, using the material sparingly.
5. As the gels are released from the syringe, they will be blended in the mixing tip and activate.

6. Place the tray into the mouth and press the gel against the teeth; remove any excess with a tissue.
7. After 30–60 minutes, remove the tray and rinse.
8. Complete the whitening treatment once a day or as directed by the dentist.
9. Do not eat, drink, or smoke while whitening or for 30 minutes after the treatment.

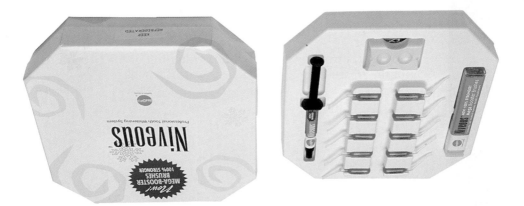

Niveous™

Professional Tooth Whitening System

New!
MEGA-BOOSTER
BRUSHES
100% STRONGER

KEEP REFRIGERATED

NICW 100% STRONGER!
Mega Booster brushes

NIVEOUS IN-OFFICE TOOTH WHITENING

MANUFACTURER:
Shofu

USE:
- Chair-side tooth whitening system
- For bleaching vital and nonvital teeth and intracoronal bleaching
- Bleaching intrinsic stains such as tetracycline stains

COMPOSITION:
- 25% hydrogen peroxide
- Approved FDA orange pigment
- Stabilizer

PROPERTIES:
- Proven to whiten teeth quickly
- Booster brushes have proprietary enhancer to optimize the whitening effect
- Convenient single-arch ampules
- Easy to use

- Long-lasting whitening effect
- Premixed gel
- Heat-activated system
- "Booster brushes" provided in the system are treated with a special oxidizing mechanism. When the booster brush is introduced to the Niveous gel, a "boosted" bleaching effect is created on the tooth.

OSHA PRECAUTIONS:

- May cause severe irritation to skin and eyes—flush with large amounts of water for 15 minutes
- Ingestion—drink lots of water and seek medical assistance

MIXING AND SETTING TIMES:

- Mixing time is 15 seconds.
- Application time is 15 minutes for each application.

DIRECTIONS:

1. Patient should have a prophylaxis treatment prior to the bleaching appointment.

2. Select and record the patient's pre-bleaching shade.
3. Remove plastic droplets and brushes from the refrigerator 15 minutes prior to the bleaching treatment to bring them to room temperature.
4. Remove the resin dam material from the refrigerator and use immediately.
5. Remove the syringe cap and place the syringe tip on the resin dam. Carefully place the dam on the gingival tissues to isolate the teeth being treated.
6. Cut the tip of the plastic droplet and dispense the gel into dappen dish or directly on the tooth.
7. Agitate the gel using the booster brush for 15 seconds in the well, and then apply to the tooth or directly on the tooth.
8. Small bubbles will appear indicating the oxidation process has begun.
9. Two applications at 15-minute periods are recommended when using a curing light that gives off heat. Use a new booster brush for each application of six teeth.

10. Using a halogen light apply to each tooth for a minimum of 2 minutes (making two passes of 1 minute each).

11. If using a high intensity laser or plasma arc light, expose each tooth for 3–5 seconds.

12. A third 15-minute application may be needed if a light source is not used with the Niveous gel.

13. Remove the bleaching gel with cotton rolls and HVE after each application followed by rinsing with water.

14. After the bleaching procedure is completed, remove the bleaching gel with cotton rolls and high-volume evacuation and then rinsing with water thoroughly.

15. Remove the resin dam material using a hand instrument. Floss may be used to remove the dam from the interproximal area.

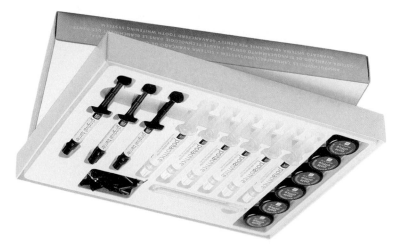

POLAOFFICE BLEACHING AGENT

MANUFACTURER:

SDI (North America) Inc.

USE:

To remove the following

- Superficial stains
- Absorbed and penetrating stains
- Age-related stains
- Conservative treatment to improve appearance
- Stains due to pulpal trauma and necrosis
- Stains from tetracycline and dental fluorosis
- Natural occurring yellow stains, chromogenic food stains, and tobacco stains

COMPOSITION:

- 35% hydrogen peroxide
- Nonhazardous balanced ingredient
- Silicone dioxide powder

- Catalyst
- Potassium nitrate

PROPERTIES:
- Simple to use
- Quick and requires minimal chair time
- Unique desensitizing properties
- Effective whitening
- Self-curing and light-curing
- Includes a gingival protectant

OSHA PRECAUTIONS:
- May be irritating to the eyes—flush immediately for 15 minutes; seek medical attention
- May be irritating to the skin—remove contaminated clothing, wash skin with soap and water; area may appear temporarily bleached white
- May cause gastrointestinal problems—do not induce vomiting drink lots of water or milk; seek medical attention

- Inhalation—remove to fresh air; if respiratory difficulties occur seek medical attention

MIXING AND SETTING TIME:
- Mixing time is 10 seconds.
- Activation time is 8 minutes for each application.

DIRECTIONS:
1. Determine and record the preoperative shade of teeth.
2. Clean the teeth with flour-based pumice.
3. Place cheek retractors and place Vaseline on lips.
4. Remove the cap from the Gingival Barrier syringe and place and secure a disposable syringe tip. Dry the teeth.
5. Using the syringe, place Gingival Barrier on both arches slightly overlapping the enamel and interproximal spaces.
6. Light-cure for 20 to 30 seconds using a fanning motion until the material is set.
7. Open the powder pot. Take one syringe of the PolaOffice, remove the cap, and place securely a disposable dispensing tip.

8. Pull back on the syringe plunger to release pressure.
9. Place the contents of the syringe into the pot and immediately mix with the brush applicator until the gel is a homogeneous mix.
10. Using the brush applicator, apply a thick layer of gel to all teeth being treated.
11. Leave the gel on the teeth for 8 minutes or you can light-cure following the manufacturer's directions.
12. Evacuate the material off the teeth using a surgical evacuating tip.
13. Repeat the application three times. A second mix needs to be completed for the third application.
14. After the last application, suction off the gel and then wash and suction the entire area thoroughly.
15. Remove the Gingival Barrier with cotton pliers by lifting it from one end.
16. Give the patient the postoperative instructions.

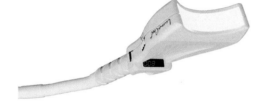

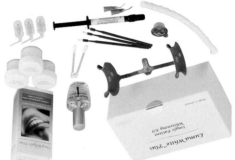

LUMA WHITE BLEACHING PASTE

MANUFACTURER:
Lumalite

USE:
- To whiten and brighten teeth
- Remove stains

COMPOSITION:
- 35% hydrogen peroxide
- Non-crystalline silica, ethanol, and proprietary trace elements

PROPERTIES:
- Achieves the best results in the least amount of time
- Convenient to use
- Everything needed is provided for in the kit.
- Low cost
- No guessing or mixing
- Protectant for gingival tissues provided

OSHA PRECAUTIONS:

- Corrosive to mucous membranes of the skin and eyes
- Eyes—may cause severe damage
- Skin—may cause irritation and burns
- Inhalation—slight nose and throat irritation
- Ingestion—corrosive to GI tract, may cause irritation, burning

MIXING AND SETTING TIME:

- Mixing time is 10 seconds.
- Activation time is 8 minutes for each of the three applications.

DIRECTIONS:

1. Determine the existing shade with the teeth moist and no overhead lighting.
2. Use flour of pumice to clean the teeth.
3. Insert cheek retractors provided in the kit.
4. For badly stained teeth apply a 5 second acid etch to the teeth.
5. Insert cotton rolls on either side of the frenum on the maxillary and mandible.

6. Thoroughly dry the teeth and the gingiva. Apply Luma Block paint on, light-curable rubber dam two teeth at a time. Light-cure the material in a slow flowing motion over the teeth. Material should be rubbery and cover all the gingival tissues.
7. Dry teeth and apply Vaseline around any exposed tissue near retractors.
8. Prepare Luma White bleach by opening the top on a catalyst jar; open one of the hydrogen peroxide premeasured ampoules by cutting the top off close to the flattened area of the tip. Dispense the material into the catalyst jar.
9. Carefully and slowly mix the material with the applicator brush for at least 10 seconds.
10. Apply the mixture to the teeth covering the cervical and incisal areas completely.
11. Insert a saliva ejector into the patient's mouth and raise the chair so the patient is sitting in an upright position.
12. Position the Full Smile Illuminator (head of the Luma whitening light) as close as possible to both arches to fully cover the area.

13. Activate the light to begin the 8 minute cycle (which can be changed if necessary).

14. When the time is completed, the light will automatically shut off.

15. Evacuate the bleaching paste from the teeth with a surgical tip on the HVE, being careful not to disturb the protective dam material.

16. Do not rinse the teeth but wipe the excess paste using a gauze pad.

17. Repeat the application of the bleaching paste two more times. Mix the bleach for each application separately.

18. After the last application, remove the bleach paste with the high-volume suction and then thoroughly rinse teeth with water and suction.

19. Remove the protective dam and cotton rolls with the explorer. Then remove the retractors.

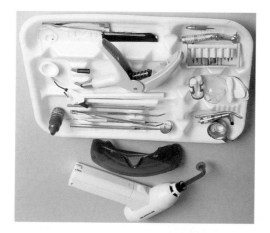

This procedure is performed by the dentist and/or the dental assistant at chairside.

EQUIPMENT AND SUPPLIES:

- Basic setup
- Air/water syringe tip, HVE, and saliva ejector
- Cotton rolls and 2 × 2 gauze sponges, applicator tips
- Rubber cup or brush
- Dri-angles
- Rubber dam setup, cotton rolls, or Garmer cotton roll holders and short and long cotton rolls
- Low-speed dental handpiece with right angle (prophy angle) attachment
- Flour of pumice or prophy paste without fluoride, or air polisher, or dry toothbrush or fissurotomy burs
- Applicators (microbrush, small cotton-tipped applicator, or syringe for etchant)

- Etchant and bonding agent or all-in-one etchant and bonding agent
- Pit & Fissure Sealant material
- Curing light
- Articulating paper and forceps
- Assorted burs, discs, and stones for reducing high spots
- PPE worn by the dental assistant

DIRECTIONS:

1. Check tooth or teeth with explorer. Polish the occlusal surface of the teeth to receive sealants. The dentist may want x-rays of the teeth to be sealed before beginning the procedure.

2. Polish the teeth using flour of pumice or a nonfluoride prophy paste with a rubber cup to clean the occlusal surfaces. (Some sealants can be used with fluoride prophy materials, check with the manufacturer before using.) An air polisher, dry toothbrush, or fissurotomy burs may also be used.

3. Once the teeth are polished, rinse and dry the teeth thoroughly. If the pits and fissures are deep, check them with an explorer and then rinse and dry again.
4. Place the chosen method of isolation—may be the dental dam, cotton rolls, or Garmer clamps.
5. Place a Dri-Angle on buccal mucosa and dry the tooth.
6. Apply the etchant using an applicator or syringe with a disposable tip to the occlusal surface, into the pits and fissures and two-thirds up the cuspid incline.
7. Etch for 15–60 seconds according to the manufacturer's directions.
8. Rinse the tooth with water, and use the evacuator tip to remove the remaining etchant and water.
9. Dry the tooth; it should have a dull chalky white appearance. If the tooth does not have this appearance, re-etch for 15–30 seconds.
10. Follow the manufacturer's directions to prepare and apply the sealant material.

11. With applicator selected, place the sealant so that it flows into the pits and fissures.
12. Light-cure the sealants, holding the curing light 2 mm directly above the occlusal surface and expose for 20 seconds on each surface.
13. Evaluate sealant with an explorer to check for voids and irregularities; repeat the process if necessary.
14. After the sealant has set, rinse, or wipe the surface with a moist cotton roll to remove the air-inhibited layer.
15. Remove the dental dam or cotton rolls.
16. Dry the teeth and place articulating paper in articulating forceps to check the bite.
17. Reduce any high spots with slow speed handpiece and burs or discs.
18. Apply fluoride to the sealed teeth.
19. Record procedure on the patient's chart.

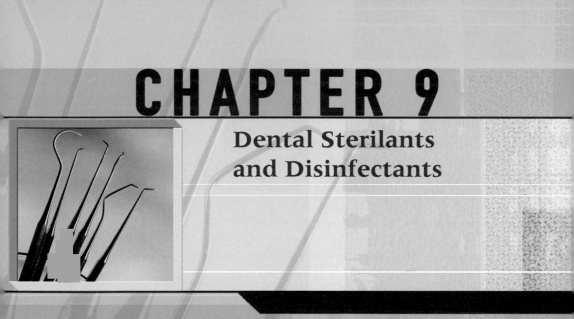

CHAPTER 9

Dental Sterilants and Disinfectants

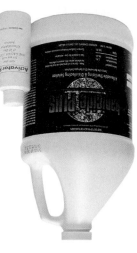

BANICIDE PLUS®

MANUFACTURER:

Pascal

USE:

- It is used for sterilization and high-level disinfection.

COMPOSITION:

- Active ingredient: 2.65% acidic, potentiated glutaraldehyde

PROPERTIES:

- Requires the addition of an activator prior to use
- Additional additives guard against corrosion.
- Effective in disinfecting impression materials and dental stone
- Mint scent
- May be used as a sterilant/high-level disinfectant for up to 28 days from initial use
- 24 degrees C
- Can be deactivated with glycide for disposal down drains
- Sterilant: 10 hours
- High-Level Disinfectant: at least 90 minutes

OSHA PRECAUTIONS:

Use appropriate PPE and follow all OSHA guidelines.

- Ingestion: It may cause irritation and possibly chemical burns of the mouth, throat, stomach, and esophagus.
- Eyes: It may cause damage to the eyes, including severe corneal injury, which may cause permanent impairment of vision. Vapors may cause stinging sensation in the eye.
- Skin: Direct solution contact may cause skin irritation or aggravation of an existing dermatitis. Skin may also turn a harmless yellow or brown color.
- Inhalation: Vapor is irritating to the respiratory tract.
- Ventilation and skin and eye protection should be used.

DIRECTIONS:

1. Open the screw lid on the gallon container and the activator.
2. Pour the activator into the plastic gallon container.

3. Place the lid back on the gallon container and move it to incorporate the activation into the entire solution.
4. Make a notation of the date that the activator was placed in the container either on the bottle or another notation close by. It is advisable to make this notation on any sterilizing or disinfecting tray that is being used.
5. The solution is ready for use for 28 days.

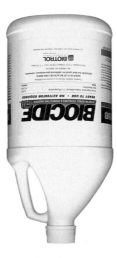

BIOCIDE G30 ™

MANUFACTURER:
Biotrol

USE:
- Used for a 30-day reusable sterilization and disinfecting solution

COMPOSITION:
- Active ingredient: 2.65% acidic glutaraldehyde

PROPERTIES:
- Ready to use
- Requires no activation
- Contains a rust inhibitor
- Active for 30 days
- Lemon scent
- Sterilizes in 10 hours
- Disinfects in 45 minutes

OSHA PRECAUTIONS:

Use appropriate PPE and follow all OSHA guidelines.

- Ingestion: Solution contact may cause irritation and possibly chemical burns.
- Eyes: Solution contact may cause damage, including severe corneal injury, which could permanently impair vision. Vapors may cause a stinging sensation in the eye.
- Skin: Direct solution contact may cause skin irritation or aggravation of an existing dermatitis. It may also cause skin to turn a harmless yellow or brown color.
- Inhalation: Vapor is irritating to the respiratory track. Ventilation and skin and eye protection should be used.

DIRECTIONS:

1. The solution is ready to use.
2. Pour the solution into the disinfecting/sterilizing tray directly from the gallon container.

3. Place notation on the container when the solution was first used. Also make a notation on the disinfecting/sterilizing tray to indicate when the solution was first used.
4. Solution is active for 30 days.

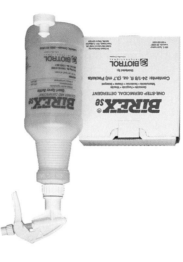

BIREX ™ SE

MANUFACTURER:
Biotrol

USE:
- Intermediate-level disinfectant, deodorizer, and cleaner for hard surfaces

COMPOSITION:
- Phenylphenol
- Phosphoric acid

PROPERTIES:
- Meets 2003 CDC guidelines for hospital disinfectants (intermediate level)
- 14-day shelf life (after mixing)
- Available in twenty-four 1/8 oz. packets and spray bottle
- Easy to store
- 10-minute disinfecting contact time
- Biodegradable

OSHA PRECAUTIONS:

Use appropriate PPE and follow all OSHA guidelines.

- Acute: Concentrate is corrosive to tissues.
- Dilution is slightly irritating to eyes.
- Concentrate is severely irritating to skin and eyes.
- It will cause an upset stomach.
- Chemical is listed as a carcinogen or potential carcinogen.

DIRECTIONS:

1. Fill water to the correct level in the quart spray bottle that comes with Birex.
2. Dispense one 1/8 oz packet into the water.
3. Label the spray bottle with the activation date.
4. Shake bottle slightly to evenly dispense the packet into the water.
5. It is ready to spray on hard surfaces for disinfecting in 10 minutes.

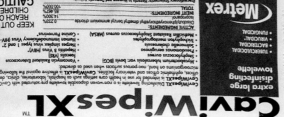

MANUFACTURER:
Metrex

USE:
- Surface disinfectant and cleaner

COMPOSITION:
- Isopropanol
- Ethylene glycol monobutyl ether

PROPERTIES:
- Disposable towelettes
- Presaturated with Cavicide Surface Disinfectant Cleaner
- Available in individually wrapped towelettes, XL (3 times larger), or a dispensing canister
- Nonwoven, nonabrasive towels
- Recommended for all nonporous surfaces
- A wall mount for the canister is available.
- 5-minute disinfectant

OSHA PRECAUTIONS:

Use appropriate PPE and follow all OSHA guidelines.

- Skin: Not considered an irritant
- Eyes: Contact with eyes can cause reversible damage.
- Inhalation: May cause low or mild irritation

DIRECTIONS:

1. Pop-up center-hinged plastic lid
2. Towelettes can be dispensed as a single sheet by tearing the perforated line or taking as many as needed before tearing the perforated line.
3. Wipe the nonporous surface for a 5-minute disinfectant.

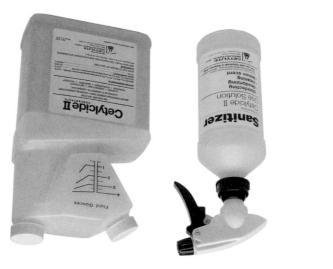

MANUFACTURER:
Cetylite Industries, Inc.

USE:
- Used as a surface disinfectant and cleaner

COMPOSITION:
- Dual quaternary ammonium compound
- Sodium carbonate
- Tergitol NP-10
- Ethylenediaminetetraacetic acid

PROPERTIES:
- EPA-registered broad-spectrum disinfectant
- Meet CDC guidelines for cleaning environmental surfaces in patient care areas
- Environmentally safe/biodegradable
- Lemon scent
- Tip and pour bottle for easy mixing

- Each quart yields 16 gallons of solution
- Biodegradable detergent with cleaning properties
- No alcohol, bleach, iodophor, phenol, or glutaraldehyde

OSHA PRECAUTIONS:

Use appropriate PPE and follow all OSHA guidelines.

- Eye: Corrosive and irritant. Prolonged contact may cause corneal burns.
- Skin Contact: Corrosive and irritant
- Ingestion: May be fatal. Burning pain, swelling in digestive tract, paralysis, circulatory shock
- Inhalation: Will cause irritation of mucous membranes, coughing, and shortness of breath
- Systemic and other effects: None reported

DIRECTIONS:

1. Fill tip and pour bottle to 1/2 oz of concentrate for one quart or 2 oz of concentrate for 1 gallon.

2. Dispense into sanitizer spray bottle that comes with the solution or obtained separately.
3. Fill the rest of the solution with water.
4. One step cleaning and disinfecting

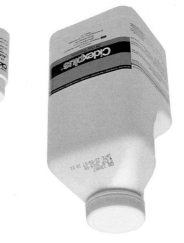

MANUFACTURER:

Advanced Sterilization Products, a Johnson & Johnson Company, division of ETHICON, Inc.

USE:

- Used for high-level disinfection

COMPOSITION:

- 3.4% alkaline glutaraldehyde solution

PROPERTIES:

- Fast-acting 28-day solution delivers a high level of disinfection in just 20 minutes at 25 degrees C.
- Packaged with an activating chemical
- Noncorrosive to instruments
- Destroys 100% of resistant *Mycobacterium tuberculosis* in 20 minutes at 25 degrees C.
- Effective in the presence of 2% organic soil
- Increased wetting and rinsing properties

- Easily discarded down office drains in accordance with state and local regulations
- Available in quart or gallon size
- Test strips available to measure the minimum effective concentration (MEC)

OSHA PRECAUTIONS:

Use appropriate PPE and follow all OSHA guidelines.

- Oral: Can irritate the tissues of the mouth, esophagus, and other tissues of the digestive system
- Eye contact: Severe irritant/corrosive to the eye
- Skin Contact: May cause skin irritation. May aggravate preexisting dermatitis
- Ingestion: This material may cause oral thrush, nausea, vomiting, epigastric distress, diarrhea, headache, fatigue, dizziness, insomnia, mental confusion, and impairment.

- Inhalation: Mist or vapors may be severely irritating to the nose, throat, and lungs.
- Ventilation and skin and eye protection should be used.

DIRECTIONS:

1. Open the container top on both the activator and the solution.
2. Pour the activator into the solution.
3. Place the top on the solution and mix slightly to incorporate the activator thoroughly.
4. Write on the bottle the date of activation and/or on the disinfecting tray to note the active date of 28 days at 25 degrees C.

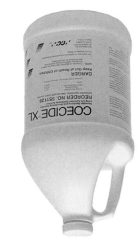

COECIDE™ XL AND COECIDE™ XL PLUS

MANUFACTURER:
GC America

USE:
- Used for sterilization, high-level disinfection, and intermediate-level disinfection

COMPOSITION:
- Coecide™ XL   2.5% alkaline glutaraldehyde
- Coecide™ XL Plus   3.4% alkaline glutaraldehyde

PROPERTIES:
- Corrosion inhibitor
- Activator included
- EPA is registered for use and reuse up to 28 days after activation.
- Can activate one quart at a time for economy
- Sterilization: 10 hours at 25 degrees C
- High-Level Disinfection: 90 minutes at 25 degrees C
- Intermediate-Level Disinfection: 10 minutes at 25 degrees C

OSHA PRECAUTIONS:

Use appropriate PPE and follow all OSHA guidelines.

- Acute and Chronic: Avoid skin contact. Repeated contact with skin may cause sensitization in some people, resulting in allergic contact dermatitis. Moderate to severe irritation to skin, eyes, and mucous membranes. Low to mild irritation by inhalation. Toxic by ingestion.
- Ventilation and skin and eye protection should be used.

DIRECTIONS:

1. Open the container top on both the activator and the solution.
2. Pour the activator into the solution.
3. Place the top on the solution and mix slightly to incorporate the activator thoroughly.
4. Write on the bottle the date of activation and/or on the disinfecting tray to note the active date of 28 days at 25 degrees C.

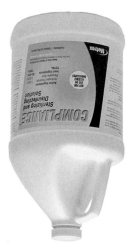

COMPLIANCE ™

MANUFACTURER:
Metrex

USE:
- It is used for high-level disinfection and sterilization.

COMPOSITION:
- Non-glutaraldehyde

PROPERTIES:
- Requires no activation
- No test strip required
- 14 day reuse
- High-level disinfectant: 15 minutes at room temperature (20 degrees C)
- Sterilant: 3 hours at room temperature (20 degrees C)

OSHA PRECAUTIONS:
Use appropriate PPE and follow all OSHA guidelines.

- Skin: Mild to moderate irritation
- Eyes: May cause irreversible tissue damage
- Inhalation: Low or mild irritation of the nose, throat, and lungs
- Ingestion: May irritate or burn mucosa membrane

DIRECTIONS:

1. Place solution in the sterilizing/disinfecting tray.
2. Instruments must be immersed into the solution.
3. Write down the date of usage on the disinfecting tray to note the active date of 14 days at 20 degrees C.

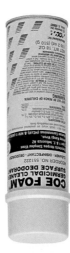

COE FOAM™ II

MANUFACTURER:
GC America

USE:
- Foaming germicidal cleaner, surface deodorant, surface disinfectant

COMPOSITION:
- Dimethyl benzyl ammonium chlorides
- Ethylbenzyl ammonium chlorides

PROPERTIES:
- Aerosol foam
- Disinfect for 10 minutes and wipe off with a clean damp cloth.
- Store away from heat or flame

OSHA PRECAUTIONS:
Use appropriate PPE and follow all OSHA guidelines.
- Causes eye and skin irritation
- Harmful if swallowed

- Product may be absorbed through intact skin
- May cause irritation to throat and gastrointestinal tract

DIRECTIONS:

1. Remove the cap, shake, spray evenly over the surface, and wipe clean.
2. For heavily soiled surfaces, allow the foam to remain for a minute before wiping.
3. To disinfect, clean as noted above and then spray a thin coat of foam over the entire surface to be disinfected.
4. Allow it to remain for at least 10 minutes and then wipe off with a clean damp cloth.

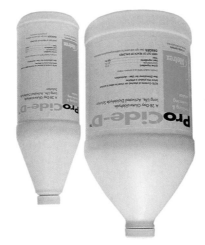

MANUFACTURER:
Metrex

USE:
- High-level disinfectant or sterilant on immersible instruments

COMPOSITION:
- Procide D® has 2.5% buffered glutaraldehyde.
- Procide D® Plus has 3.4% buffered glutaraldehyde.

PROPERTIES:
- Attains an alkaline pH of between 7.5 and 8.5
- Active up to 28 days at temperature of 25 degrees C
- Sterilization: 10 hours at 25 degrees C
- Disinfection: 90 minutes at 25 degrees C

OSHA PRECAUTIONS:
Use appropriate PPE and follow all OSHA guidelines.

- Skin: Mild to moderate irritation
- Eye: Direct contact with eyes can cause irritation
- Ingestion: Toxic
- Inhalation: Low or mild irritation

DIRECTIONS:

1. Place solution in the sterilizing/disinfecting tray.
2. Instruments must be immersed into the solution.
3. Write down the date of usage on the disinfecting tray to note the active date of 28 days at room temperature (25 degrees C).

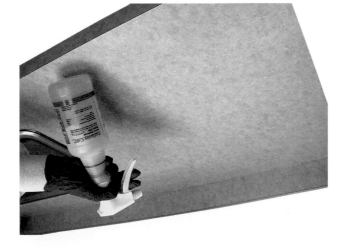

PROSPRAY™ C-60

MANUFACTURER:
Certol International, LLC.

USE:
- Surface disinfectant

COMPOSITION:
- Active ingredients: o-phenylphenol and o-benzyl-p-chlorophenol

PROPERTIES:
- 1/2 oz unit-dose tubes for mixing
- Does not stain or bleach hard surfaces
- Lemon scent
- Spray bottle has nozzle with 3 adjustable settings (off, spray, and stream)
- Meets all CDC guidelines for surface disinfection
- Approved for 60-day use
- Available in wipes

OSHA PRECAUTIONS:

Use appropriate PPE and follow all OSHA guidelines.

Effect of overexposure:

- Swallowing: Irritation of the mouth, throat, and digestive tract
- Skin contact: May cause mild irritation
- Inhalation: May cause mild irritation
- Eye contact: May cause irritation

DIRECTIONS:

1. Fill 16 oz ProSpray C-60 bottle with room temperature water to the fill line.
2. Add 1/2 oz of ProSpray C-60 to filled spray bottle using unit dose or measuring cup.
3. This is when the 60-day shelf life begins. Note this on the container.
4. Disinfect and clean surfaces using spray nozzle or optional squirt cap

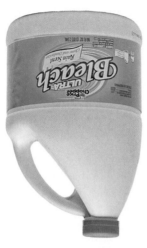

SODIUM HYPOCHLORITE (BLEACH)

USE:
- Intermediate-level surface disinfection

COMPOSITION:
- 5.25% sodium hypochlorite "household bleach"

PROPERTIES:
- Works within 10 minutes
- Unstable; must be mixed daily
- Corrosive to metals
- Harmful to clothing

OSHA PRECAUTIONS:
Use appropriate PPE and follow all OSHA guidelines.
- Irritation or damage to skin and eyes may occur.
- Use in a well-ventilated room. Avoid inhalation.

- Do not mix with other chemicals.
- If swallowed, mucosal and gastric damage will occur; call a physician.

DIRECTIONS:

1. Mix 1 cup of sodium hypochlorite with one gallon of water.
2. Place the solution into a spray bottle or onto a sponge.
3. Allow it to remain for at least 10 minutes and then wipe off with a clean damp cloth.
4. Take extra care not to get solution on clothing.
5. Solution should be disposed of at the end of each day.

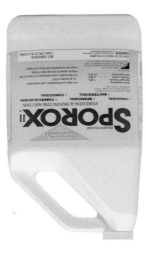

SPOROX II

MANUFACTURER:
Sultan Healthcare

USE:
- Sterilizing and high-level disinfecting solution

COMPOSITION:
- Active ingredient: hydrogen peroxide 7.5%

PROPERTIES:
- Ready to use; no mixing or activation required
- No noxious odors
- Oxidizes away dental debris and contaminants
- High-level disinfecting   30 minutes (20 degrees C/68 degrees F)
- Sterilization   6 hours (20 degrees C/68 degrees F)
- May be reused up to 28 days
- Test vials available

OSHA PRECAUTIONS:

Use appropriate PPE and follow all OSHA guidelines.

- Corrosive to eyes
- May be harmful or fatal if swallowed
- Do not get in eyes, on skin, or on clothing
- Use safety glasses and gloves.

DIRECTIONS:

1. Place the solution in sterilizing/disinfecting tray. No activation is required.
2. Instruments must be immersed into the solution for 6 hours.
3. Write down the date of usage on the disinfecting/sterilizing tray to note the active date of 21 days at room temperature (20 degrees C/68 degrees F).

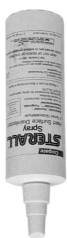

MANUFACTURER:
Colgate

USE:
- Sterilizing and high-level disinfectant

COMPOSITION:
- Active ingredient
- Sterall® Plus   Glutaraldehyde 3.4%
- Sterall®   2.65% potentiated glutaraldehyde

PROPERTIES:
- Sterall®
  - One-year shelf life
  - Contains corrosion inhibitor
  - Lemon scent
  - No activator needed
  - 30-day reuse life
  - Used for sterilization and high-level disinfection

- Sterall® Plus
- Light mint scent
- Corrosion inhibitor
- 28-day reuse life
- Activator required for sterilization solution

OSHA PRECAUTIONS:

Use appropriate PPE and follow all OSHA guidelines.

- Acute and Chronic: Avoid skin contact. Repeated contact with skin may cause sensitization in some people, resulting in allergic contact dermatitis. Moderate to severe irritation to skin, eyes, and mucous membranes. Low to mild irritation by inhalation. Toxic by ingestion.
- Ventilation and skin and eye protection should be used.

DIRECTIONS:

1. Spray bottle is ready for use as a disinfectant/decontaminate cleaner.
2. Spray on inanimate surfaces and operatory equipment.
3. Allow it to remain for at least 10 minutes and then wipe off with a clean damp cloth.

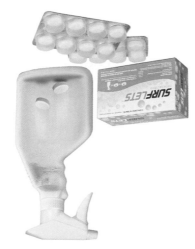

SURFLETS DISINFECTANT TABLETS

MANUFACTURER:
Sultan Healthcare

USE:
* Intermediate-level disinfectant
* Disinfectant for impression materials

COMPOSITION:
* Sodium dichloroisocyanurate, dihydrate
* Sodium bisulfate

PROPERTIES:
* Sixteen tablets in blister packaging
* Neutral pH, bromine-based formula
* Not corrosive
* Effective for 7 days
* No mixing—add 2 tablets to 32 oz of water
* Saves storage space
* Mild lemon fragrance

OSHA PRECAUTIONS:

Use appropriate PPE and follow all OSHA guidelines.

- Eye Contact: Slightly irritating, avoid contact with eyes.
- Skin Contact: Slightly irritating, avoid contact with skin.
- Inhalation: No data available
- Ingestion: No data available

DIRECTIONS:

1. Place 2 tablets into spray bottle with 32 oz of water.
2. This solution is effective for 7 days so it can be made weekly; if not, the day the water and tablets were combined should be noted on the spray container.
3. Spray nonporous surfaces and/or impression materials.
4. Allow it to remain for at least 5 minutes and then wipe off with a clean damp cloth or rinse off the impression materials.

PROCEDURE: DISINFECTING SURFACES IN THE DENTAL OPERATORY

This procedure is performed by the dental assistant in the dental operatory.

EQUIPMENT AND SUPPLIES:

- Disinfecting solution in spray bottle is mixed and ready.
- 4 × 4 gauze
- Wiping cloth
- Small utility carry tote to hold or transport items if desired

DIRECTIONS:

1. Review MSDS sheet for the solution.
2. Wear appropriate PPE.
3. Wash hands and pull on utility gloves.
4. Bring the equipment and supplies to the operatory.
5. Have a routine procedure established for disinfection to ensure that nothing is missed. All surfaces need to be sprayed and

cleaned first, then wiped to remove debris. The surfaces are then sprayed a second time and the solution is left on surfaces for a designed time according to the manufacturer's directions.

6. Spray on the disinfectant and leave it for the correct time to accomplish disinfection.
7. Rewipe all surfaces after the time has lapsed.

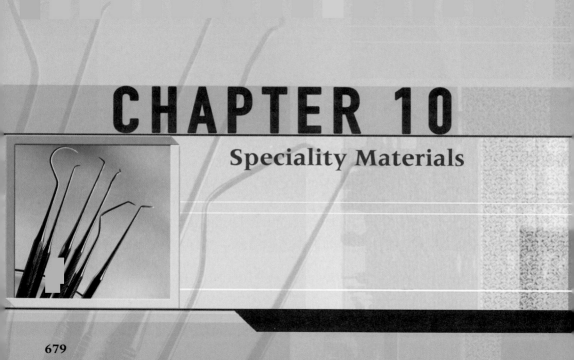

CHAPTER 10

Speciality Materials

APEXIT ENDODONTIC SEALER/CEMENT

MANUFACTURER:
Ivoclar Vivadent

USE:
- Permanent obturation of root canals

COMPOSITION:
- Base and Activator: Calcium hydroxide, calcium oxide, inorganic fillers, colophony, disalicylate

PROPERTIES:
- High bio-compatibility
- Low water solubility
- Mixes easily
- High radiopaque
- Non-shrinking material
- Can be used with all obturating systems

- Flows easily into canals and adapts to the walls of the root canals
- Comes in automix syringes for easy handling

OSHA PRECAUTIONS:
- Eye irritation: Flush with water for 10 to 15 minutes
- Skin irritation: Wash with soap and water
- Ingestion: No hazards anticipated from swallowing small amount during incidental or normal handling
- Inhalation: Remove to fresh air

MIXING AND SETTING TIME:
- Automix syringes requiring no mixing
- Working time is approximately 3 hours.

DIRECTIONS:
1. Remove the cap from the automix syringe by turning it a 1/4 turn counterclockwise.

2. Insert the mixing tip by pushing down until the notch of the tip is aligned with the double-push syringe.
3. Secure the mixing tip in place by gripping the colored base and turning a 1/4 turn clockwise.
4. The double-push syringe contains predosed amounts of Apexit Plus activator and base, which are automatically mixed and dispensed when the two materials are extruded.
5. The material is placed into the canal with a Lentulo spiral or an Intra Oral Root Canal tip.

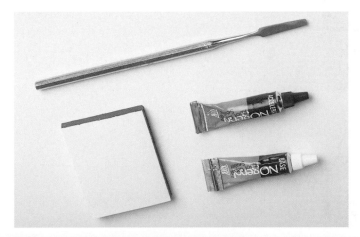

MANUFACTURER:
GC America

USE:
- Root canal sealer

COMPOSITION:
- Base: salicylic acid
- Catalyst: zinc oxide, vegetable oil, barium sulfate, and bismuth oxychloride

PROPERTIES:
- Biocompatible
- No eugenol
- Radiopaque
- Sets quickly in the mouth
- Two-paste system that is easy to mix and use
- Long-working time
- Allows time for placement and manipulation of material

- Adheres to dry surface
- Seals and adapts to the tooth surface well
- Low solubility

OSHA PRECAUTIONS:
- Eye and skin irritation possible with prolonged exposure
- Ingested:
  - Base—induce vomiting and seek medical attention
  - Catalyst—drink several glasses of water
- Inhalation: remove to fresh air and seek medical attention

MIXING AND SETTING TIME:
- Mixing time is 10 to 15 seconds
- Setting time is 7 minutes in the mouth

DIRECTIONS:
1. The dentist prepares the root canal according to routine root canal treatment.
2. Prepare and pass paper points to dry the canal.

3. Extrude equal lengths of each paste on a paper pad. Approximately 3/4 of an inch of each paste.
4. Spatulate for 10 to 15 seconds until mix is uniform in color and consistency.
5. Nogenol Root Canal Sealer has a long working time on the paper pad, but once placed in the mouth it will set in about 7 minutes.
6. Prepare a spreader or other endodontic instrument to place the sealer.
7. Prepare the gutta percha points or silver points to be coated with the sealer.

SEALAPEX XPRESS NON-EUGENOL ROOT CANAL SEALER

MANUFACTURER:

SybronEndo

USE:

- Seal the root canal after the root canal treatment

COMPOSITION:

- Isobutyl salicylate, silicone dioxide, bismuth trioxide, titanium dioxide pigment
- Base: N-ethyl toluene, sulfonamide resin, silicone dioxide, zinc oxide, and calcium hydroxide

PROPERTIES:

- Non-eugenol
- Non-irritating
- No manual mixing required
- Stimulates hard tissue formation
- One to one syringe ratio

OSHA PRECAUTIONS:

- May be irritating to the eyes and skin.
- Inhalation may cause drowsiness. Remove to the fresh air.
- If ingested, consult a physician.

MIXING AND SETTING TIME:

- No mixing required

DIRECTIONS:

1. Remove the cap from the automix syringe by turning it a 1/4 turn counterclockwise.
2. Insert the mixing tip by pushing down until the notch of the tip is aligned with the double-push syringe.
3. Secure the mixing tip in place by gripping the colored base and turning a 1/4 turn clockwise.

4. The automix syringe contains pre-dosed amounts of Sealapex Xpress catalyst and base, which are automatically mixed and dispensed with the two materials extruded.
5. The material is placed into the canal with a Lentulo spiral or an Intra Oral Root Canal tip.

ROOT CANAL SEALER

MANUFACTURER:
Pulpdent

USE:
- Permanent root canal filling material
- Used to seal root canals in both primary and permanent dentition

COMPOSITION:
- Liquid: eugenol
- Powder: zinc oxide

PROPERTIES:
- Tissue compatible
- Bacteriostatic
- Radiopaque
- Used with all permanent filling techniques
- Expands slightly upon setting to assure a positive seal

- Resorbs with roots of primary teeth
- Insoluble
- Flows through 30 gauge needles for root apex placement
- Slight overfills resorb in 10 to 12 months

OSHA PRECAUTIONS:
- Eye and skin irritation possible
- Should not be ingested

MIXING AND SETTING TIME:
- Mixing time is approximately 15 to 30 seconds
- Setting time is approximately 5 to 10 minutes

DIRECTIONS:
1. After the root canal has been opened, enlarged, and cleaned by the dentist, a Pulpdent Pressure syringe tip is selected.
2. Measure the powder and liquid to maintain a 1:1 ratio.

3. Fluff the powder bottle before using and then with the designated scoop, dispense 3 scoops of powder on to the pad. Be sure to level the scoop of powder.
4. Drop 3 drops of liquid on the pad and mix until a uniform, putty-like consistency.
5. Material will be pliable enough to form a homogeneous mass.
6. Fill the hub of the syringe with the Pulpdent Root Canal Sealer thick mix to prepare the syringe for use.

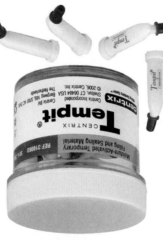

TEMPIT MOISTURE-ACTIVATED TEMPORARY FILLING AND SEALING MATERIAL

MANUFACTURER:
Centrix

USE:
- For sealing access cavities during root canal treatment appointments

COMPOSITION:
- Calcium sulfate and zinc oxide, glycol, ethyl methacrylate polymer, barium sulfate, and silica

PROPERTIES:
- No mixing and no mess
- Sets in minutes
- Easy to remove
- Non-eugenol formula

OSHA PRECAUTIONS:
- Eyes: Flush with copious amounts of water and seek medical attention
- Skin irritation possible: Wash with soap and water
- Ingested: N/A
- Inhalation: N/A

MIXING AND SETTING TIME:
- There is no mixing
- Setting time: 5 minutes or less

DIRECTIONS:
1. Remove the cap from the syringe.
2. Place the tip securely on the end of the syringe.
3. Squeeze the syringe with slow steady pressure to ensure the syringe is functional.
4. Dispense a small amount on the pad then inject into the moist canal.

5. Tamp down with a moist instrument and dismiss the patient.
6. On the patient's return appointment, use an explorer to remove Tempit material.

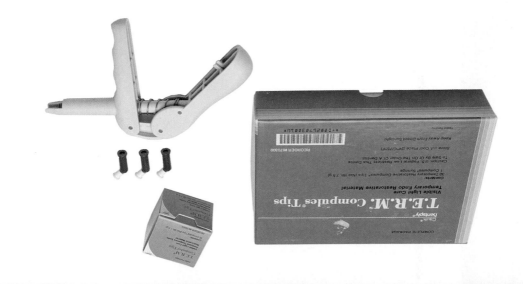

T.E.R.M. TEMPORARY RESTORATIVE MATERIAL

MANUFACTURER:
Dentsply/Mailefer

USE:
- Temporary restorative material in the root canal access orifice

COMPOSITION:
- Aluminum oxide, silica amorphous, silica crystalline, urethane dimethacrylate resin

PROPERTIES:
- Light-cured material
- Firm restoration
- Easy-to-place Compule tips
- Superior moisture-free seal
- Quick to remove with bur or hand instrument
- Creamy paste

OSHA PRECAUTIONS:

- May cause skin irritations
- Persons susceptible to methacrylates, acrylics, and urethanes may develop allergic response.
- Dermal redness or irritation may occur, and several allergic responses may cause difficulty in breathing.
- Should not be ingested
- May cause mild respiratory irritation

MIXING AND SETTING TIME:

- No mixing required
- Light-cure to set

DIRECTIONS:

1. Select a Compule tip and Compule syringe.
2. Snap the Compule tip into the syringe making sure it is secure.

3. Remove the cap and squeeze the handle until T.E.R.M. Temporary Restorative Material starts to flow.
4. Place the material into the access orifice, compact the material, and then light-cure for 20 seconds.

BUCKLEY FORMO CRESOL

MANUFACTURER:
Sultan Healthcare

USE:
- Devitalize and sterilize infected pulp chambers and canals

COMPOSITION:
- 35% Cresol
- 19% Formaldehyde
- 17.5% Glycerin

PROPERTIES:
- Slightly less irritating to periapical tissues
- Lower content of formaldehyde

OSHA PRECAUTIONS:
- Eye contact—flush with plenty of running water

- Skin irritation possible—wash with soap and water and remove contaminated clothing
- Ingestion—quickly give 3 or more glasses of milk or water
- Inhalation—remove to fresh air and have qualified person restore and/or support breathing with oxygen

MIXING AND SETTING TIME:
- No mixing is required

DIRECTIONS:
1. Clean the tooth and root canal.
2. Use a cotton tip applicator or cotton pellets to apply the Formo Cresol.
3. Place the applicator in the Formo Cresol, remove excess liquid, and place in the canal.

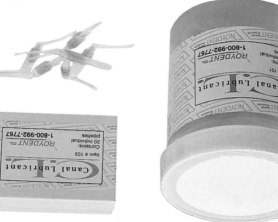
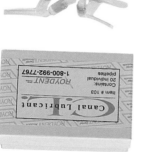

Courtesy of Roydent Dental

C.L. CANAL LUBRICANT

MANUFACTURER:
Roydent Dental

USE:
- Chelates root canal walls
- Aids in enlarging the root canals
- Assists in instrumentation by lubricating the canals

COMPOSITION:
- 17% ethylenediaminetetraacetic acid in aqueous gel

PROPERTIES:
- Lubricates the canal
- Softens calcifications in the root canals

OSHA PRECAUTIONS:
- Inhalation: none
- Eyes: may cause transient irritation

- Skin: nonirritating
- Ingestion: none expected with this product with normal conditions of use

MIXING AND SETTING TIME:
- There is no mixing.
- There is no setting time.

DIRECTIONS:
1. C.L. Canal Lubricant comes in pipettes for easy dispensing.
2. With the material in pipettes it can be placed directly in the canal or a reamer or file can be used to place the lubricant into the canal.
3. Holding the pipette, cut the tip off. The pipette is then squeezed for dispensing.

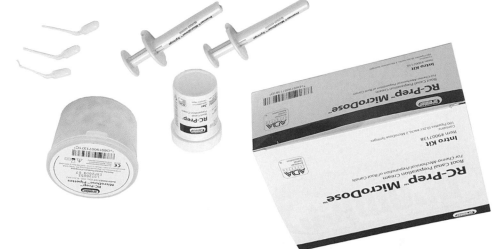

RC-PREP ROOT CANAL PREPARATION CREAM

MANUFACTURER:
Premier

USE:
- Chemo-mechanical preparation for root canals

COMPOSITION:
- Glycol, urea peroxide, and EDTA in special water soluble

PROPERTIES:
- Removes calcifications from the root canal
- Lubricates the canal for efficient instrumentation
- Used with apex locators for reliable readings
- Allows for efficient use of reamers and files
- Prevents instruments from binding
- Easy to use
- Also come in a microdose form

OSHA PRECAUTIONS:

- Skin: There may be irritation and redness. Remove contaminated clothing and wash with soap and water.
- Eyes: There may be pain and redness and eyes may water. Vision may blur. Rinse with water for 15 minutes and seek medical assistance.
- Ingestion: There may be soreness and redness in the mouth and throat. Nausea and stomach pain may occur. Wash out mouth with water, give water to drink, and seek medical assistance.
- Inhalation: There may be irritation in the throat and a feeling of tightness in the chest. Remove from exposed area.

MIXING AND SETTING TIME:

- There is no mixing.

DIRECTIONS:

1. RC-Prep comes in jars, pumps, or syringes.
2. With the material in the jars and pumps, a reamer, file, or root canal filler is used to place the RC-Prep into the canal. Dispense

a small amount of the RC-Prep on a pad and then coat the reamer, file, or root canal filler with the material.

3. With the syringe, the material is placed directly into the canal with the tip of the syringe.

4. When the material reacts with the sodium hypochloride, it lifts the debris from the canal.

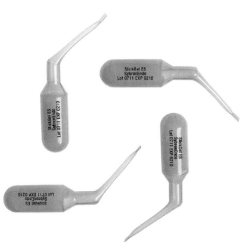

SLICKGEL ES ROOT CANAL LUBRICATING AGENT

MANUFACTURER:
SybronEndo

USE:
- Aids in the negotiation of root canals

COMPOSITION:
- Ethylenediamine, tetraacetic acid, urea peroxide, proplyene glycol, and polyethylene glycol

PROPERTIES:
- High effervescent action that produces vigorous bubbling
- Chemically removes the smear layer
- Helps prevent blockage during shaping and cleaning
- Lubricates the canal that aids in negotiation of the root canals
- Aids in softening calcifications in the root canal
- Easy to use
- Comes in Micro Dose Polytubes that do not require disinfection after each use, reducing cross-contamination

- Smooth solution not grainy

OSHA PRECAUTIONS:

- **Eyes:** Flush with water for 15 minutes.
- **Skin:** Wash with soap and water thoroughly.
- **Swallowing:** Drink two glasses of water and seek medical attention.

MIXING AND SETTING TIME:

- There is no mixing or setting time.

DIRECTIONS:

1. SlickGel comes in Micro Dose Polytubes.
2. When the dentist is ready, the assistant cuts the end of a unidose polytube and passes it to the dentist.
3. The dentist places the tip of the polytube into the root canal and squeezes.
4. At the end of the procedure the polytube is thrown away.

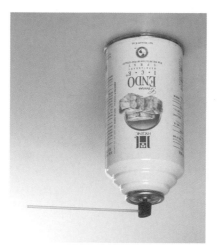

ENDO-ICE

MANUFACTURER:
Coltene/Whaledent

USE:
- To test pulp vitality

COMPOSITION:
- Tetrafluoroethane

PROPERTIES:
- Fast and easy method for testing pulp vitality
- Much colder than ice or ethyl chloride
- Spearmint scent
- Directional spray extension

OSHA PRECAUTIONS:
- After inhalation: Get fresh air.
- After skin contact: Wash with water for 15 minutes.
- After eye contact: Flush with water for 15 minutes.

- After swallowing: Drink water to dilute. Do not induce vomiting.
- If irritation persists, contact a physician with all of the above.

MIXING AND SETTING TIME:

- No mixing or setting times

DIRECTIONS:

1. Place spray extension into the cap securely.
2. Have cotton tip applicator or cotton pellet ready.
3. Spray the applicator or pellet and hand to the dentist to apply to the tooth.

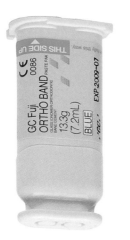
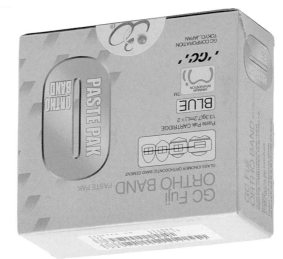

FUJI ORTHO LC CEMENT

MANUFACTURER:
GC America

USE:
- Orthodontic light-cured adhesive that bonds to metal and porcelain brackets and metal bands

COMPOSITION:
- Liquid: Polyacrylic acid, hydroxyethyl methacrylate
- Powder: Alumino-silicate glass

PROPERTIES:
- Low sensitivity to moisture
- Use with or without etching
- Significant fluoride release and recharge
- Available in both powder/liquid and capsules
- Prevents caries—no decalcification
- High success rate
- Easy to use and clean up

OSHA PRECAUTIONS:

- Eyes: May be irritating to the eyes, rinse for 15 minutes
- Skin: May be irritating to the skin, wash for 15 minutes
- Ingestion: Do not induce vomiting. Drink large volumes of water.
- Inhalation: Powder—Remove to fresh air. Drink water to clear throat and blow nose to remove dust particles.
- If irritation develops, seek medical attention with all of the above.

MIXING AND SETTING TIME:

- Total mixing time is 20 to 25 seconds.
- Working time is 3 minutes from start of mix.

DIRECTIONS:

1. Clean the surface with nonfluoridated prophy paste and water.
2. Rinse thoroughly with water.

3. Dispense a few drops of GC Fuji Ortho Conditioner into a well. Dip a gauze or sponge into the conditioner and apply to the bonding surfaces of the teeth for 20 seconds. Rinse.
4. Enamel bonding surfaces must be moist.
5. Tap the powder and then dispense one level scoop with designated scoop onto a paper pad.
6. Holding liquid vertical, gently squeeze to dispense 2 drops onto the paper pad.
7. Divide the powder into two parts. Bring one part of powder into all the liquid and mix for 10 seconds. Bring the second portion of powder into the mix and mix for 10 to 15 seconds until smooth, creamy, and uniform.
8. Fuji Ortho cement is ready to use.

HELIOSIT ORTHODONTIC

MANUFACTURER:
Ivoclar Vivadent

USE:
- Permanently cementing orthodontic brackets—metal or ceramic

COMPOSITION:
- Paste of dimethacrylate, bis-GMA, silicone dioxide, catalyst, and stabilizers

PROPERTIES:
- Light-curing material
- Highly translucent
- No dosing or mixing required
- High strength bond

OSHA PRECAUTIONS:

- May be irritating to the eyes. Flush with water.
- May be irritating to the skin. Wash with soap and water.
- Ingestion: No hazard anticipated from swallowing small amounts incidental to normal handling
- Inhalation: Remove to fresh air.
- If irritation develops, seek medical attention with all of the above.

MIXING AND SETTING TIMES:

- No mixing required
- Light-cured for a total of 40 seconds

DIRECTIONS:

1. Clean the surface thoroughly.
2. Isolate with cotton rolls and blown air.
3. Apply etchant to the tooth according to manufacturer's instructions. Usually etchant is applied for 30 to 60 seconds.

4. Rinse and dry the area thoroughly. The tooth surface should look chalky.
5. Remove the cap from the Heliosit Orthodontic cement and place a small amount on the bracket according to the bracket manufacturer's instructions. The cement may also be placed on a paper pad and using an instrument placed on the bracket.
6. Replace the cap.
7. Light-cure the bracket once placed for 20 seconds from the cervical and 20 seconds from the incisal.

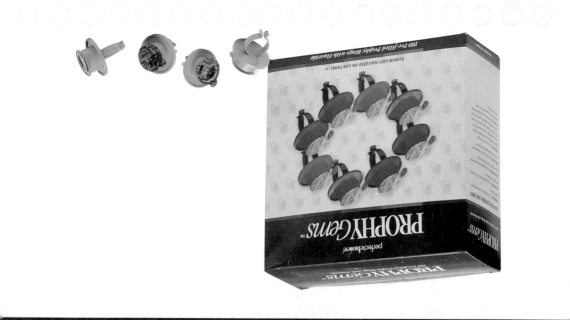

PERFECT CHOICE PROPHY GEMS PROPHY PASTE

MANUFACTURER:
Biotrol

USE:
- Cleaning paste to remove deposits and stains from the teeth

COMPOSITION:
- Blend of cleaning and polishing agents
- Sodium fluoride and sodium saccharine

PROPERTIES:
- Removes tough stains
- Low splatter paste
- Variety of grits
- Contains fluoride
- Rinses easily
- Variety of flavors
- Rings are color-coded by flavor.

- Lip for thumb hold ring in place
- Ring is comfortable and secure on finger.

OSHA PRECAUTIONS:

- Eyes: Direct contact will cause irritation.
- Skin: Prolonged contact will cause irritation.
- Ingestion: Contains sodium fluoride, do not swallow.

MIXING AND SETTING TIMES:

- None

DIRECTIONS:

1. Determine the grit to use by evaluating the amount of hard and soft deposits a patient has.
2. Select the grit and flavor.
3. Remove the foil seal from the Prophy Gems.
4. Remove the prophy paste with a prophy angle and cup to begin the polish.

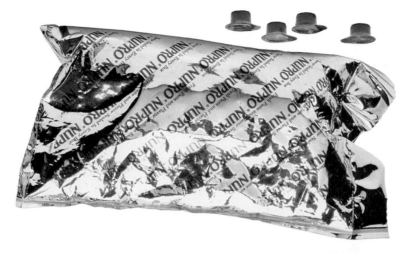

NUPRO PROPHY PASTE CUPS VARIETY
PAK WITH FLUORIDE

MANUFACTURER:
Dentsply Professional

USE:
- Prophy paste to remove soft and hard deposits from the teeth

COMPOSITION:
- Blend of polishing and cleaning agents
- 1.23% fluoride ion

PROPERTIES:
- Excellent stain removing and polishing
- Variety of grits and flavors
- Spatter-free formula
- Rinses easily and completely
- Always consistent
- Comes in unidose cups, jars, and variety paks
- With and without fluoride

OSHA PRECAUTIONS:

- Skin: not applicable
- Eyes: Flush with water. If irritation persists, contact a physician.
- Ingestion: Give copious amounts of water or milk and call a physician.
- Inhalation: not applicable

MIXING AND SETTING TIMES:

- Does not apply

DIRECTIONS:

1. Each cup contains enough prophy paste to complete one patient.
2. Remove foil from prophy cup.
3. If finger grip is used, place prophy cup in finger grip and secure.
4. Attach rubber cup to prophy angle.
5. Place the rubber cup into the prophy paste while running the angle at low speeds.
6. To avoid overheating the tooth, always keep enough prophy paste in the rubber cup to be used on the teeth.

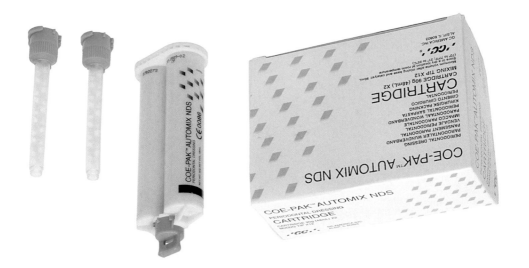

COE-PAK AUTOMIX NDS PERIODONTAL DRESSING

MANUFACTURER:
GC America

USE:
- Non-eugenol surgical and periodontal dressing

COMPOSITION:
- Vegetable oil, zinc oxide, mineral oil, magnesium oxide, chlorodimethyl phenol ethanol, methanol, and petrolatum

PROPERTIES:
- No burning sensation
- No unpleasant taste
- No strong odor
- Protection to tissues
- Promotes cleanliness and healing
- Resilient hardness to resist fracture or breakage
- Smooth cohesive mix

- Automix or two-paste system
- Material won't stick to gloves.

OSHA PRECAUTIONS:

- Eyes: May be irritating to the eyes. Flush for 15 minutes.
- Skin: May be irritating to the skin. Wash for 15 minutes with soap and water.
- Ingestion: Drink several glasses of water.
- Inhalation: Remove to fresh air. Drink water to clear throat and blow nose to remove dust particles.
- If irritation develops, seek medical attention with all of the above.

MIXING AND SETTING TIME:

- Ready to use in 3 minutes
- Hard and fast set ready in 1 minute

DIRECTIONS:

1. Place an automix cartridge into a GC cartridge dispenser II.
2. Remove the cap from the cartridge and place a mixing tip.

3. Dispense the required amount of material on a paper pad.
4. Using a spatula, form the material into a cylindrical shape.
5. Lightly lubricate your fingers with Vaseline, lanolin, cold cream, or water to test the mix for thickness.
6. Automix material will lose its tackiness in about 30 seconds, whereas the two-paste mix should lose its tackiness in 2 to 3 minutes.
7. Automix will be workable for 8 minutes; two-paste mix can be worked for 10 minutes.
8. Form into ropes. Material is extremely cohesive. Place in patient's mouth.

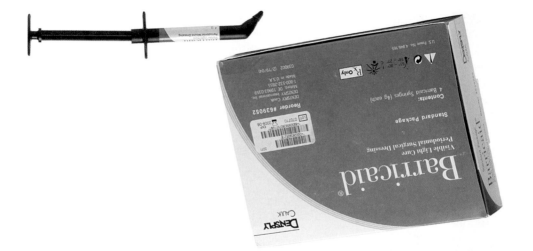

BARRICAID VLC SURGICAL PERIODONTAL DRESSING

MANUFACTURER:
Dentsply Caulk

USE:
- Light-cured surgical periodontal dressing
- Protection for periodontal surgical sites during the healing process

COMPOSITION:
- Dimethacrylate resins

PROPERTIES:
- Control over the setting time of the material
- Light-cured
- Designed for direct and indirect placement
- Material forms a nonbrittle, elastic protective cover.
- Is tasteless
- Tinted pink with translucent qualities

OSHA PRECAUTIONS:

- **Eyes:** Rinse with open eyes for several minutes under running water.
- **May be irritating to the skin:** Immediately wash with soap and water and rinse thoroughly.
- **Ingestion:** If symptoms persist, contact a physician.
- **Inhalation:** Remove to fresh air.

MIXING AND SETTING TIME:

- No mixing is required.
- Light-cured for 10 seconds per tooth on both buccal and lingual sides

DIRECTIONS:

Barricaid Periodontal Dressing can be applied directly or indirectly.

1. **Direct Technique:** Using sterile gauze, dry the buccal or lingual surfaces adjacent to the surgical site.

2. Remove the cap from the syringe and begin dispensing the material at the juncture of the cervical 1/3 of the teeth and the margin of the surgical site.
3. Indirect Technique: Using sterile gauze, dry the buccal or lingual surfaces adjacent to the surgical site.
4. Place a thin layer of lubricant on a paper pad. Remove the cap from the syringe and dispense the amount needed.
5. Place a light layer of lubricant on your gloved hand and roll the material off the pad ready to be placed.
6. Once placement is completed, light-cure for 10 seconds the buccal and lingual of each tooth
7. Check for uncured material with a blunt instrument or explorer.

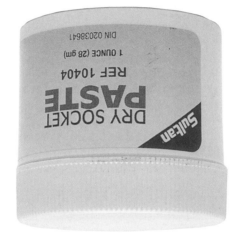

DRY SOCKET PASTE

MANUFACTURER:
Sultan Healthcare

USE:
- To treat Alveolitis (dry socket)

COMPOSITION:
- Gualacol, balsum peru, eugenol, 1.6% chlorobutanol

PROPERTIES:
- Easy to use
- Instant pain relief
- Effective treatment
- Only one treatment needed

OSHA PRECAUTIONS:
- May be irritating to the eyes: Lifting eyelid, flush with large amounts of running water for 15 minutes.
- May be irritating to the skin: Remove contaminated clothing and wash area with soap and water.

- Irritating to the respiratory system: Remove patient to fresh air.
- If ingested, contact a physician.

MIXING AND SETTING TIME:

- No mixing
- Material remains in the socket for 3 to 5 days.

DIRECTIONS:

1. Socket is prepared.
2. Remove the lid from the paste.
3. Remove the amount necessary to fill the socket.
4. Place material into the socket with a flat-bladed instrument and pack into place.
5. Tamp down to cover exposed bone.
6. Material remains in the socket for 3 to 5 days.
7. Paste washes out gradually as the socket heals.

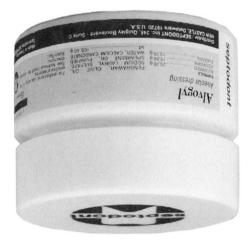

ALVOGYL

MANUFACTURER:
Septodont

USE:
- Dry socket treatment
- Post-extraction dressing

COMPOSITION:
- Eugenol, butamben, and iodoform

PROPERTIES:
- One-step dressing
- Rapidly alleviates pain
- Soothing effect throughout healing process
- Fibrous consistency for good adherence during healing
- Analgesic action
- Anesthetic action
- Anti-microbial action

OSHA PRECAUTIONS:

- May be irritating to the eyes and skin
- Irritating to the respiratory system: Remove to fresh air.
- If ingested, contact a physician.

MIXING AND SETTING TIME:

- No mixing required

DIRECTIONS:

1. Socket or surgical site is prepared.
2. Remove the lid from the paste.
3. Remove the amount necessary to fill the socket.
4. Place material into the socket with a flat-bladed instrument and pack into place.
5. Tamp down to cover the exposed bone.
6. Material remains in the socket as the socket heals.

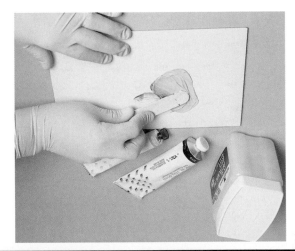

This procedure is performed by the dentist and/or the dental assistant at chairside.

EQUIPMENT AND SUPPLIES:
- Basic setup
- Air/water syringe tip, HVE, and salvia ejector
- Cotton rolls and 2 × 2 gauze sponges
- Periodontal dressing catalyst and base tubes
- Paper pad—large
- Large spatula or tongue depressor
- Lubricant (Vaseline, lanolin, cold cream, water)
- Instrument to contour dressing (spoon excavator)
- PPE worn by the dental assistant

DIRECTIONS:
After the hemorrhaging is controlled, the patient's lips are coated lightly with a lubricant. The dental assistant prepares the periodontal dressing for application as follows before placement:

1. Extrude equal lengths of paste from the catalyst and base tubes onto the paper pad.
2. Spatulate for 30 to 45 seconds until the mix is of uniform color.
3. Using the spatula, form the paste into a cylindrical shape.
4. Lightly lubricate gloved fingers with Vaseline, cold crème, lanolin, or water to test the mixed paste for tackiness. It should be ready in 2 to 3 minutes.
5. After 2 to 3 minutes the dressing paste can be handled. Remove the cylindrical shape from the paper pad and mold into the diameter and length needed to place over surgical site.
6. The dressing paste can be worked for 10 to 15 minutes. This gives the dentist or dental assistant enough time to place and secure the dressing on the buccal and lingual surfaces of the surgical site.
7. The dressing is secured around the most posterior tooth and then pressed interproximally on the buccal surfaces. This procedure is repeated on the lingual surfaces.

8. Once the dressing is placed, it is evaluated for effectiveness and comfort for the patient. Adjustments are completed.
9. Give home care instructions to the patient and dismiss.

INDEX

3. Seat the mixing tip completely into the open holes on the MixStar cartridge.
4. Secure the mixing tip by sliding the locking mechanism into locked position over the mixing tip.
5. Insert the cartridge into the mixing unit.
6. Turn on the mixing unit and as the material is dispensed, flow the material into the tray keeping the tip in the material and not trapping air into the material.
7. Insert the tray into the patient's mouth and hold time noted according to material used.
8. Remove from patient's mouth, rinse, and disinfect.
9. Wait 30 minutes and pour the impression.

HYDROCOLLOID-REVERSIBLE HYDROCOLLOID IMPRESSION MATERIAL

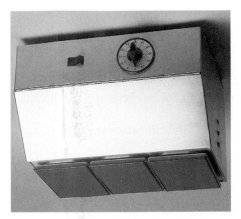

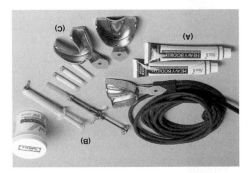

Courtesy of Van R

MANUFACTURER:
Van R

USE:
- Crown and bridge impressions
- Inlay and onlay impressions

COMPOSITION:
- Made from water and the ocean's agar

PROPERTIES:
- Wetness
- Small amounts of blood and saliva do not affect the accuracy of the impression.
- Available in syringe and tubes
- Must be used with a Hydrocolloid machine

OSHA PRECAUTIONS:

- Principal hazardous components—none
- No occupational control measures needed

MIXING AND SETTING TIME:

Acculoid, Lavender, Extra Strength
  5 minute temper at 110°F/43°C
  7 minute cooling in the mouth with room temperature water
  Stores 5 days once liquefied

AgarLoid, Blue, Fast Tempering
  4 minute temper at 110°F/43°C
  5 minute cooling in the mouth with room temperature water
  Stores 5 days once liquefied

Slate, Gray, High Strength
  5 minute temper at 110°F/43°C
  5 minute cooling in the mouth with room temperature water
  Stores 4 days once liquefied

Qwik, Chocolate
  3 minute temper at 110°F/43°C
  3 minute cooling in the mouth with room temperature water
  Stores 3 days once liquefied

DIRECTIONS:

After the tray is selected, PPE in place, and the patient is prepared for procedure:

1. Remove the tube from the storage compartment of the hydrocolloid conditioner. Fill the water-cooled tray and place in the tempering bath.
2. Set the timer to the correct time for tempering according to the material being used.
3. After the time has concluded, remove the syringe material that is in the cartiloid and place it into the syringe. Attach a hydrocolloid syringe tip to the cartiloid and apply pressure to the syringe to expel a small amount of material while taking to

the operator to use. This ensures that the material does not set up in the tip.

4. Remove the impression from the tempering bath and place a 2 × 2 over the material to dry off the top surface. Attach the tubing to the impression and hand it to the operator to place into the mouth.

5. After the impression is seated in the mouth, attach the tubing to the water source and start the water flowing. Set the timer.

6. Remove from patient's mouth, rinse and pour immediately.

USE:
- Used to make impressions prior to newer materials being developed
- Mounting casts

COMPOSITION:
The composition is produced by heating mineral gypsum in an open kettle at temperatures of 110 degrees to 120 degrees C. This produces crystals that are slender and porous and relatively soft.

PROPERTIES:
- Beta-hemihydrate
- Reproduction detail poor
- Formatted for remounting casts
- Fast-setting plaster
- Requires more water to wet each surface
- Calcinated in an open kettle method

- Takes more water to incorporate the mixture
- After the mixture dries, the areas where the water was now become air spaces.
- Weaker than stone or type II model or laboratory plaster.
- White in color

OSHA PRECAUTIONS:

- Eye and skin irritation possible
- Should not be ingested
- May cause respiratory tract irritation if inhaled

MIXING AND SETTING TIMES:

- Ratio: 60 ml of water to 100 grams of powder
- Set in 4–5 minutes

DIRECTIONS:

1. Use a rubber bowl and a stiff spatula
2. Press against the bowl; don't whip (causes more air to be incorporated into mixture).

3. Mixing should take about 1 minute.
4. Over-spatulating will cause a breakdown of crystals and soft spots in the model.

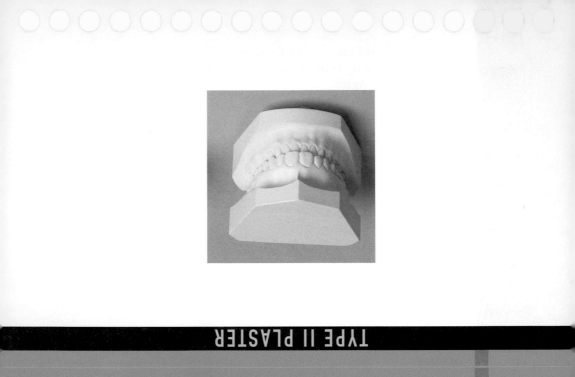

TYPE II PLASTER

USE:
- Versatile formulation for multiple applications
- Study models
- Opposing models
- Repairing casts
- Mounting models and casts

COMPOSITION:
The composition is produced by heating mineral gypsum in an open kettle at temperatures of 110 degrees to 120 degrees C. This produces crystals that are slender and porous and relatively soft.

PROPERTIES:
- Beta-hemihydrate
- Requires more water to wet each surface
- Calcinated in an open kettle method
- Takes more water to incorporate the mixture

- After the mixture dries, the areas where the water was now become air spaces.
- Weaker than stone, stronger than type I model or laboratory plaster
- White in color

OSHA PRECAUTIONS:

- Eye and skin irritation is possible.
- Should not be ingested
- May cause respiratory tract irritation if inhaled

MIXING AND SETTING TIMES:

- Ratio: 50 ml of water to 100 grams of powder
- Working time 5–7 minutes
- Initial set loses glossiness and does not flow.
- Final set can no longer be penetrated.
- Set in 15–30 minutes for separation.

DIRECTIONS:

1. Use a rubber or disposable bowl and a stiff spatula.
2. Press against the bowl; don't whip (causes more air to be incorporated into mixture).
3. Place the mixture on a vibrator to allow the air bubbles to rise to the top surface.
4. Mixing should take about 1 minute.
5. Consistency should be one where the spatula can cut through the mixture and it stays to the sides without changing position.
6. It will appear like whipped cream with a smooth, creamy texture.
7. Over-spatulating will cause a breakdown of crystals and soft spots in the model.

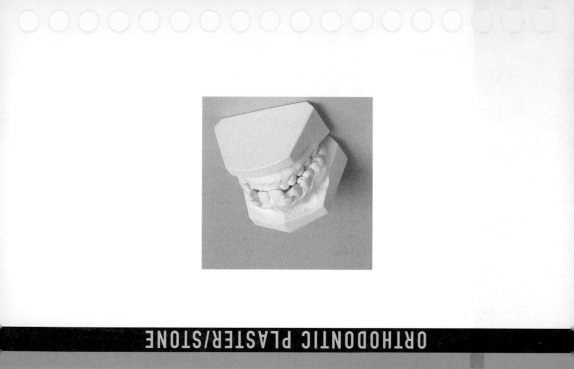

ORTHODONTIC PLASTER/STONE

USE:

- For making orthodontic casts (models)

COMPOSITION:

Type II Plaster and Type III Laboratory Stone Mixed Together

PROPERTIES:

- Mixture of type II plaster and type III stone
- Purchased as orthodontic stone-premixed
- Sets harder than models made from type II
- Denser than ordinary plasters
- Easy to trim
- White in color

OSHA PRECAUTIONS:

- Eye/face protection
- Skin protection to prevent drying or irritation of hands
- Respiratory protection—NIOSH-approved dust mask or filtering face-piece is recommended in poorly ventilated areas.

MIXING AND SETTING TIMES:

- Ratio: 40 ml of water to 100 grams of powder
- Working time 5–7 minutes
- Initial set loses glossiness and does not flow.
- Final set can no longer be penetrated.
- Set in 15–30 minutes for separation

DIRECTIONS:

1. Use a rubber or disposable bowl and a stiff spatula.
2. Press against the bowl; don't whip (causes more air to be incorporated into mixture).
3. Place the mixture on a vibrator to allow the air bubbles to rise to the top surface.
4. Mixing should take about 1 minute.
5. Consistency should be one where the spatula can cut through the mixture and it stays to the sides without changing position.

6. It will appear like whipped cream with a smooth, creamy texture.
7. Over-spatulating will cause a breakdown of crystals and soft spots in the model.

MAGIC WHITE

MANUFACTURER:
Dental Vencura Madespa

USE:
- Orthodontic models

COMPOSITION:
Is produced by driving off water of crystallization under an elevated steam pressure at about 125 degrees C.

PROPERTIES:
- Bright white
- Stronger than plaster
- Quick setting
- Comes in plastic bucket with closing lid

OSHA PRECAUTIONS:

- Skin contact: May cause dry skin, discomfort, and irritation
- Inhalation—breathing dust may be harmful—use mask
- Ingestion: Small quantities not known to be harmful but large amounts may cause an obstruction

MIXING AND SETTING TIMES:

- Ratio: 26 ml of water to 100 grams of powder
- Working time—7 minutes
- Initial set—7 minutes
- Final set—7 1/2 minutes

DIRECTIONS:

1. Use a rubber or disposable bowl and a stiff spatula or a vacuum mixing device.
2. Press against the bowl; don't whip (causes more air to be incorporated into mixture).

3. Place the mixture on a vibrator to allow the air bubbles to rise to the top surface.
4. Mixing should take about 1 minute.
5. Consistency should be one where the spatula can cut through the mixture and it stays to the sides without changing position.
6. It will appear like whipped cream with a smooth, creamy texture.
7. Over-spatulating will cause a breakdown of crystals and soft spots in the model.

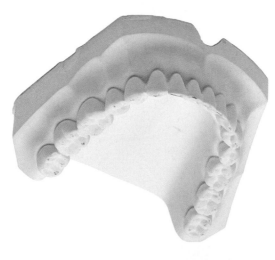

TYPE III LABORATORY STONE

USE:
- Diagnostic casts
- Working casts
- Models for partial and full dentures
- Articulating
- Flasking

COMPOSITION:
Is produced by driving off water of crystallization under an elevated steam pressure at about 125 degrees C

PROPERTIES:
- Calcinated by steam under pressure
- More strength than Type I and Type II
- Usually yellow, green, or blue in color
- Referred to as alpha-hemihydrate

OSHA PRECAUTIONS:

- Skin contact: May cause dry skin, discomfort, and irritation
- Inhalation—breathing dust may be harmful—use mask
- Ingestion: Small quantities not known to be harmful but large amounts may cause an obstruction

MIXING AND SETTING TIMES:

- Ratio: 30 ml of water to 100 grams of powder
- Working time 5–7 minutes
- Initial set loses glossiness and does not flow.
- Final set—no longer can be penetrated
- Set in 15–30 minutes for separation

DIRECTIONS:

1. Use a rubber or disposable bowl and a stiff spatula or a vacuum mixing device.
2. Press against the bowl; don't whip (causes more air to be incorporated into mixture).

3. Place the mixture on a vibrator to allow the air bubbles to rise to the top surface.
4. Mixing should take about 1 minute.
5. Consistency should be one where the spatula can cut through the mixture and it stays to the sides without changing position.
6. It will appear like whipped cream with a smooth, creamy texture.
7. Over-spatulating will cause a breakdown of crystals and soft spots in the model.

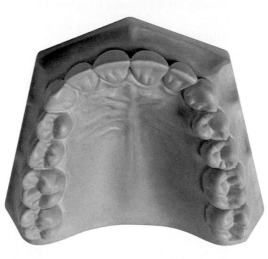

TYPE IV DIE STONE

USE:
- For making dies (A die is a positive replica of the prepared tooth made from stone.)
- In making a cast or model where strength is important

COMPOSITION:
Is commonly produced by dehydration in an autoclave in the presence of sodium succinate or in a kettle with a 30% calcium chloride solution.

PROPERTIES:
- Extra strong, extra hard
- High strength, low expansion
- Hard, smooth surfaces when poured
- Calcinated by autoclaving in the presence of calcium chloride.
- Modified alpha-hemihydrate that is referred to as die stone
- Stronger and more dense than Type I, II, and III
- Normally supplied in colors rose, peach, light blue, or light buff

OSHA PRECAUTIONS:

- Skin contact: May cause dry skin, discomfort, and irritation
- Inhalation—breathing dust may be harmful—use mask
- Ingestion: Small quantities not known to be harmful but large amounts may cause an obstruction

MIXING AND SETTING TIMES:

- Ratio: 24 ml of water to 100 grams of powder (normally supplied in premeasured packets)
- Working time 5–7 minutes
- Initial set loses glossiness and does not flow.
- Final set—no longer can be penetrated
- Set in 15–30 minutes for separation

DIRECTIONS:

1. Use a rubber or disposable bowl and a stiff spatula or a vacuum mixing device.
2. Press against the bowl; don't whip (causes more air to be incorporated into mixture).

3. Place the mixture on a vibrator to allow the air bubbles to rise to the top surface.
4. Mixing should take about 1 minute.
5. Consistency should be one where the spatula can cut through the mixture and it stays to the sides without changing position.
6. It will appear like whipped cream with a smooth, creamy texture.
7. Over-spatulating will cause a breakdown of crystals and soft spots in the model.

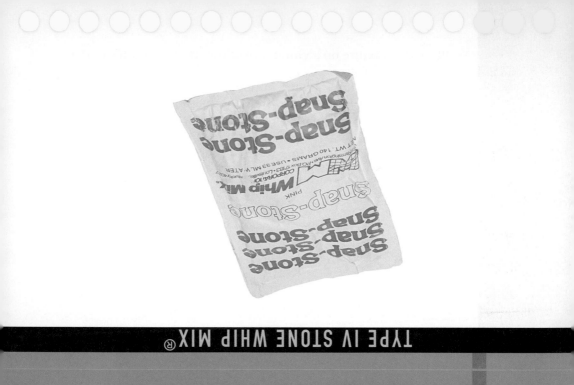

MANUFACTURER:
Whip Mix Corporation

USE:
- Bleaching trays
- CAD-CAM restorations
- For making dies (A die is a positive replica of the prepared tooth made from stone.)
- In making a cast or model where strength is important
- Implants, porcelain, and inlay/only cases

COMPOSITION:
Is commonly produced by dehydration in an autoclave in the presence of sodium succinate or in a kettle with a 30% calcium chloride solution

PROPERTIES:
- Exceptionally fast setting
- Resin reinforced for maximum strength

- Minimum expansion
- Thixotropic (liquid that flows easily under mechanical forces), yet highly stackable for easy sculpting
- Provides high definition, detailed models
- Tough, durable, nonbrittle
- Enhanced abrasion resistance
- Great stability over time
- No change or very little change in expansion
- Stronger and more dense than Type I, II, and III

OSHA PRECAUTIONS:
- Skin contact: May cause dry skin, discomfort, and irritation
- Inhalation—breathing dust may be harmful—use mask
- Ingestion: Small quantities not known to be harmful but large amounts may cause an obstruction

MIXING AND SETTING TIMES:
- Ratio: 23 ml of water to 100 grams of powder (normally supplied in pre-measured packets)

- Working time: 60–90 seconds
- Setting time: 2 minutes

DIRECTIONS:

1. Use a clean, flexible rubber, disposable or plastic bowl.
2. Use the proper ratio of water to powder. Measure room temperature water into mixing bowl.
3. Add powder to liquid.
4. Use a clean, stiff spatula and spatulate at a rate of 120 RPM for 60 seconds until a smooth and uniform mix is achieved. If using a vacuum mixer, the recommended time is 15 seconds.

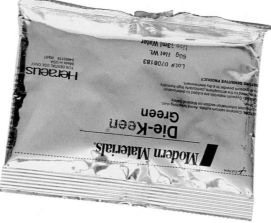

TYPE V DIE STONE

MANUFACTURER:
Modern Materials

USE:
- Where a really strong die model is needed
- Implants, inlays, crown and bridge dies

COMPOSITION:
Is commonly produced by dehydration in an autoclave in the presence of sodium succinate or in a kettle with a 30% or more calcium chloride solution. Additional refining and increased pressure of the powder by grinding results in a denser stone.

PROPERTIES:
- High strength
- High expansion
- Recently approved by the American Dental Association (ADA)
- Optimum expansion for dies and crown and bridge work

- Ultra fine
- Flows easily during vibration

OSHA PRECAUTIONS:

- Skin contact: May cause dry skin, discomfort, and irritation
- Inhalation—breathing dust may be harmful—use mask
- Ingestion: Small quantities not known to be harmful but large amounts may cause an obstruction

MIXING AND SETTING TIMES:

- Ratio: 21 ml of water to 100 grams of powder (normally supplied in premeasured packets)
- Initial set—10–13 minutes
- Final set—no longer can be penetrated

DIRECTIONS:

1. Use a clean, flexible rubber, disposable or plastic bowl.
2. Use the proper ratio of water to powder. Measure room temperature water into mixing bowl.

3. Add powder to liquid.
4. Use a clean, stiff spatula and spatulate at a rate of 120 RPM for 60 seconds until a smooth and uniform mix is achieved. If using a vacuum mixer, the recommended time is 15 seconds.

MODERN MATERIALS® STATSTONE

MANUFACTURER:

Modern Materials/Heraeus Kulzer

USE:

- When speed and precision are needed for fabricating:
  - Custom trays
  - Mouth guards
  - Vacuum-formed splints
  - Denture repairs

COMPOSITION:

Is commonly produced by dehydration in an autoclave in the presence of sodium succinate or in a kettle with a 30% or more calcium chloride solution. Additional refining and increased pressure of the powder by grinding results in a denser stone.

PROPERTIES:

- Fast and accurate
- High early compression strength
- Low expansion
- Well suited for bleaching application
- Available in light pink

OSHA PRECAUTIONS:

- Skin contact: May cause dry skin, discomfort, and irritation
- Inhalation—breathing dust may be harmful—use mask
- Ingestion: Small quantities not known to be harmful but large amounts may cause an obstruction

MIXING AND SETTING TIMES:

- Ratio: 23 ml of water to 100 grams of powder (normally supplied in premeasured packets)
- Initial set—2 minutes
- Ready for removal from the impression in just 5 minutes

DIRECTIONS:

1. Use a clean, flexible rubber, disposable or plastic bowl.
2. Use the proper ratio of water to powder. Measure room temperature water into mixing bowl.
3. Add powder to liquid.
4. Use a clean, stiff spatula and spatulate at a rate of 120 RPM for 60 seconds until a smooth and uniform mix is achieved. If using a vacuum mixer, the recommended time is 15 seconds.

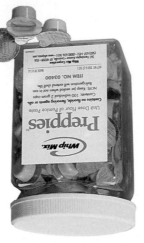

PUMICE

MANUFACTURER:
Whip Mix Corporation

USE:
- Polishing dental appliances such as provisionals, dentures, partials, and bridges

COMPOSITION:
Volcanic silica manufactured as a loose abrasive. Flour of pumice is extremely fine.

PROPERTIES:
Available in grades:

- Pumice, Flour
- Pumice, Fine
- Pumice, Medium
- Pumice, Coarse
- Pumice, X-Coarse

Specially ground for fast cutting without scratching or grooving

MIXING AND SETTING TIMES:

- Used with water and a lathe to smooth the appliance
- No mixing required

DIRECTIONS:

1. Remove pumice from canister without contamination of other pumice.
2. Place about 1/3 cup into the slash pan of the lathe.
3. Add water to the pumice to make a putty-like material.
4. Wet the rag wheel and place it on the lathe.
5. If the appliance has not been sterilized, the rag wheel and the splash pan will need to be sterilized/disinfected and the pumice discarded. The EPA issued guidelines for dental issues in 1999 for caring for dental pumice.
6. Place the pumice on the appliance in the area that requires smoothing. Using the rag wheel of the lathe, smooth the area.
7. The pumice needs to be fed into the area that needs polishing during the rotation of the rag wheel.

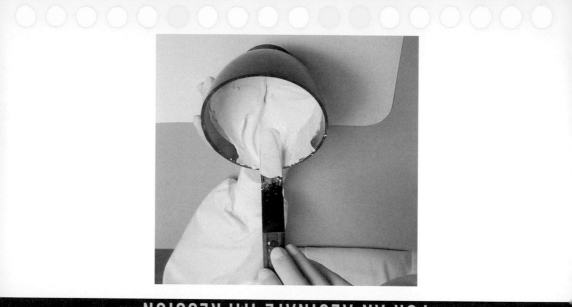

PROCEDURE: MIXING THE PLASTER
FOR AN ALGINATE IMPRESSION

This procedure is performed by the dental assistant in the dental laboratory.

EQUIPMENT AND SUPPLIES:

- Spatula, metal with rounded end and stiff, straight sides
- Two flexible rubber mixing bowls
- Scale
- Type II plaster (100 grams)
- Gram measuring device
- Water measuring device
- Vibrator with paper or plastic cover on the platform
- Room temperature water
- Alginate impression (disinfected) PPE worn by assistant

DIRECTIONS:

1. Measure 50 ml of room temperature water into one of the flexible mixing bowls.
2. Place the second flexible mixing bowl on the scale and set the dial to zero. This allows the plaster powder to be weighed.

3. Weigh out 100 grams of plaster in the second rubber bowl.
4. Add the powder from the second bowl to the water of the first bowl. Placing the water in first allows for all the powder to become incorporated into the mixture. Allow several seconds for the powder to dissolve into the water.
5. Use the spatula to slowly mix the particles together. The initial mixing should be completed in 20 seconds. The total mixing procedure should take about 1 minute.
6. Turn on the vibrator to medium or low speed.
7. Place the rubber bowl on the vibrator platform, pressing lightly.
8. Rotate the bowl on the vibrator to allow the air bubbles to rise to the top surface. The mixing and vibrating should be completed within a couple of minutes. The mixture is ready if the spatula can cut through it and it stays to the sides without changing positions. It will appear like whipped cream with a smooth, creamy texture. Another way to check whether the powder/water ratio is in correct ratio is to place a spoonful on the spatula and turn it upside down—if the material remains in place, the mixture is ready.

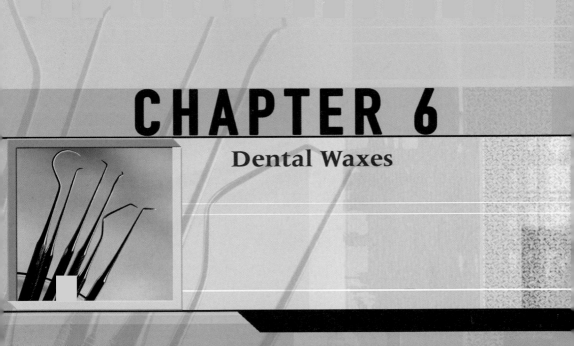

CHAPTER 6

Dental Waxes

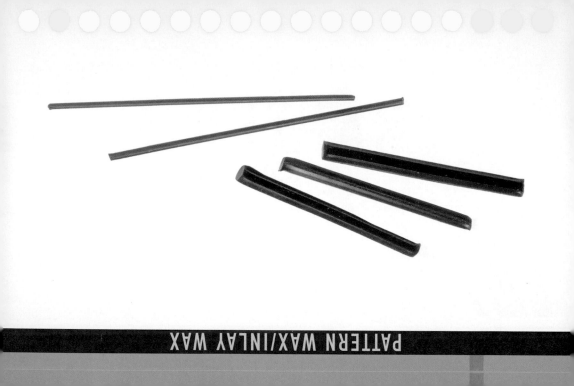

PATTERN WAX/INLAY WAX

USE:

- To make a wax pattern of the restoration (crown or bridge) to be made

COMPOSITION:

- 40–60% paraffin wax
- 10% gum dammar
- 25% carnauba wax
- 10% ceresin wax
- 5% beeswax

Note: Composition will vary from manufacturer to manufacturer.

PROPERTIES:

- It is a hard wax used in crown and bridge construction.
- Comes in dark blue, green, or purple rods or sticks about 7.5 cm long and 6 mm in diameter (3 inches long and 1/4 inch in diameter).
- Used on a die to make a replica of the final restoration.

- **Type I** is used for direct techniques (establishing the initial form of the tooth in the oral cavity) and it is a little softer.
- **Type II**, most often used in the dental laboratory, is used for indirect techniques where the wax pattern is carved on the die (stone model).

OSHA PRECAUTIONS:

- Nonhazardous at room temperature
- If exposed to melted wax, fumes may cause irritation.
- Direct contact with molten material may cause injury. Flush area with cold water.

DIRECTION:

The wax is melted and applied to the die (a positive replica of the prepared tooth made of stone) layer by layer until the contacts, margins, anatomy, and occlusion are correct. It will resemble the final crown or bridge that is being made.

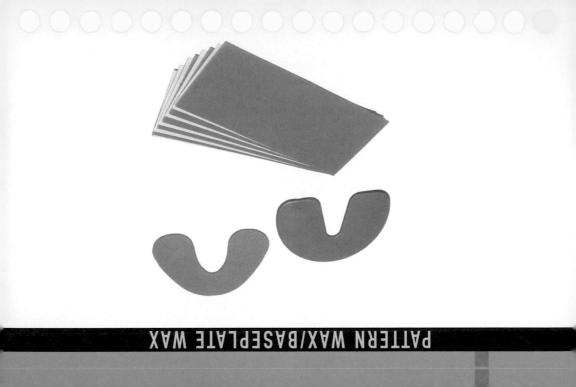

USE:

- Construction of the baseplate tray to establish the vertical dimension in the initial arch for a denture or partial

COMPOSITION:

- 80% ceresin
- 12% beeswax
- 2.5% carnauba
- 5% natural or synthetic resins

Note: Composition will vary from manufacturer to manufacturer.

PROPERTIES:

- Available in three types:
  - Type I—a softer baseplate wax that is used for building contours and veneers
  - Type II—a medium wax used for patterns to be tried into the mouth in temperate climates (most commonly used)
  - Type III—a harder wax to be used in the mouth in tropical weather or when extra hardness is required

- Carves without chipping
- Boils out cleanly
- Pliable
- Shaded to resemble gum tissue (pink color)
- Unlimited shelf life
- Available in shapes that resemble the dental arches
- The Type II can be heated with warm water or a flame and used for taking a bite.

OSHA PRECAUTIONS:

- Nonhazardous at room temperature
- If exposed to melted wax, fumes may cause irritation.
- Direct contact with molten material may cause injury. Flush area with cold water.

DIRECTIONS:

1. Dental baseplate wax can be heated with a torch and adapted easily to a stone model of the edentulous arch.

2. It should be adapted closely and the excess trimmed with a wax spatula or blade. The softer wax is tough yet pliable all-purpose wax.
3. The margins of the wax should be made smooth to the touch due to the fact that it is going to be reinserted into the patient's mouth.

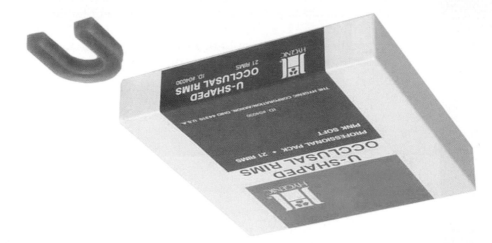

PATTERN WAX—OCCLUSAL RIMS OR BITE BLOCKS

USE:
- It is a softer wax block that is attached to the baseplate wax that is used in the construction of the tray to establish the vertical dimension in the initial arch for a denture or partial.

COMPOSITION:
- Hazardous components—none
- Less than 10% petroleum hydrocarbons and additives

PROPERTIES:
- Can be shaped at room temperature
- Some types come with a recessed base to aid in adapting it to the baseplate.
- Can be adapted to fit any arch
- Can be easily heated to set the denture teeth into it
- U-shaped
- Pink in color
- Soft but not sticky
- Referred to as either occlusal rim or a bite block

OSHA PRECAUTIONS:

- Nonhazardous at room temperature
- Above its melting point, wax becomes liquid and flows more readily as its temperature increases. Use special handling with hot liquid wax.

DIRECTIONS:

1. Adapt the U-shaped wax arch to the baseplate on the stone model of the edentulous arch.
2. Heat the recessed base of the arch and stick it to the baseplate.
3. Ensure the two are adapted securely.
4. Smooth the area where the two waxes (baseplate and bite rim) come together.

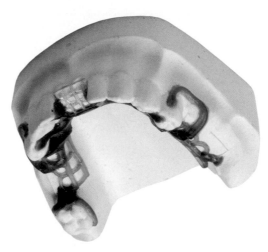

USE:

- It is used to fabricate the pattern for the metal framework for removable partial dentures and other similar structures.

COMPOSITION:

- The composition is the same as inlay waxes but contains reduced amounts of hard waxes and increased amounts of beeswax.

PROPERTIES:

- Easily trimmed with sharp knife
- Has a smooth, glossy surface after gently flaming
- Sold in:
  - Thin sheets
  - Preshaped like completed metal framework or clasps
  - Square sheets
  - Long thin strips

OSHA INFORMATION:

- Nonhazardous at room temperature

- Above its melting point, wax becomes liquid and flows more readily as its temperature increases. Use special handling with hot liquid wax.

DIRECTIONS:

1. Use the wax and place it on the stone model where the metal framework will be after fabrication.
2. Attach all wax on the model and secure it together.
3. Use a flame to smooth areas and obtain the glossy finish needed.

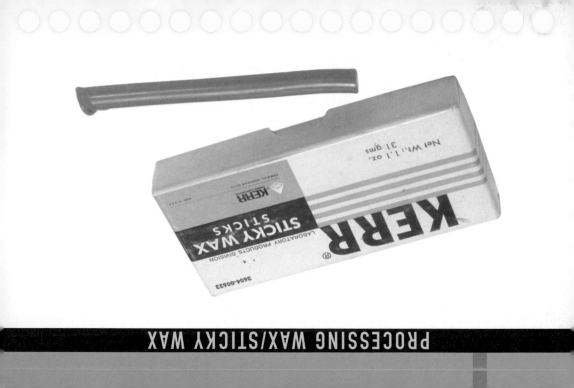

USE:
- It is used to adhere two materials together for fabrication or repairs. It has many uses.

COMPOSITION:
- Hazardous components—none
- Less than 10% petroleum hydrocarbons and additives

PROPERTIES:
- Brittle wax at room temperature but when melted with a flame it is sticky
- Adheres to a number of surfaces such as metal, stone, plaster, tooth structure, etc.
- Will fracture rather than flow if deformed
- Comes in a number of colors—usually orange or dark red
- Normally available in sticks
- Melting temperature 136 degrees F (58 degrees C)

OSHA PRECAUTIONS:

- Nonhazardous at room temperature
- Above its melting point, wax becomes liquid and flows more readily as its temperature increases. Use special handling with hot liquid wax.

DIRECTIONS:

1. Place the two materials that need to be adhered together.
2. Heat the tip of the sticky wax stick with a flame.
3. Touch the end that has been heated to the items that need to be attached and the sticky wax will set up rapidly.
4. The wax will change to a milky color when set.

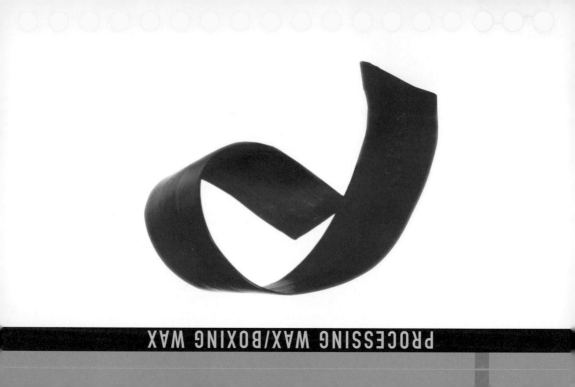